The Body Engineer

ISBN- 978-1542341660

www.bodyengineering.com

To those that said It never could be done without the use of harmful drugs, thank you for motivating me. I would like to give a special dedication to my grandpa, Randy Martin, my father, Bryan Loyd, and my High School wrestling coach, Kirk Moore for giving me the mentally strength to fight through any adversity or challenge.

Table of Contents

About the Author

Hi, my name is Shane and I believe in fitness. Not like your personal trainer (been there, done that) or your local gymnastics team. I actually believe in fitness. Fitness is the most powerful drug on the planet; it makes a person want to better themselves in all aspects of life. It makes a person want to stick to a plan to perfect their body and their health. When one is healthy, they are on their A game. They can wear the dress they want, they have confidence, they can pick up on women at the clubs, climb a mountain, and most importantly, they can set a good example.

I will tell you I am not in this for the money. If I was in it for the money I would become a Dr. and advise you to take this pharmaceutical drug or lab test so I can get a $500$3,000 kickback to pay for my Mercedes. I've tried to chase the money as a fitness sales advisor. I made over six-figures, but I HATED it. Why? Because I was given a manuscript to sell off of, and I knew the information was BS. If you have a personal trainer, it is most likely that they don't practice what they preach. Yes, there are a slight few that really care about their clients, but for the most part you are just another stepping stone. My goal is to impact as many lives as possible by educating them on the various correct methods of natural fitness and or bodybuilding. My biggest accomplishment will be the day that I am known as the guy who helped hundreds of millions of people.

What's my main drive, you ask? My grandpa died at the age of 67 and the other at 47. They both practiced unhealthy eating practices and did not exercise. I literally watched my grandpa die at 67; he just gave up and I begged him to get out of his bed, but he just wouldn't do it. He loved the hell out of me, but he could barely breathe, he was overweight, and he was on a load of pharmaceutical drugs. After that incident, at the age of 20, I committed my life to nourishment and to find the healthiest way to live possible. I've done my research and have tried every diet in the book. I'm here to tell you the truth about what it takes.

-My Journey

I will begin this book by giving you a little background on myself. At the age of 12, I was an overweight chubby kid. I would do your typical push-ups and sit ups and bike riding, but I got made fun of. I didn't fit in with the popular kids. I knew I had to make a change and I had to make it fast. I scrapped up enough money to buy myself a weight set from doing concrete with my father. Like many of you reading, I had very little knowledge on how to lift weights or where to start. But that didn't matter, because I had a goal.

I would lift in my backyard every morning before middle school and then high school came around. I made the varsity football team as a freshman. Yes, I was that kid for once. I was kind of popular. Let me tell you, it felt great! I was the biggest guy at my school. Just from lifting on my own while everyone else was out getting stoned or drinking. I knew from this day on hard work does pay off in the long run.

I always worked out and ate semi-healthy, but I worked out for sports like wrestling and football. Looking back today, my high school and college coaches were blinded. They knew practically nothing about nutrition and or building muscle. They were coaching our team under what they thought was the correct way to build muscle and nourish our bodies. I would push myself to the max and I would work out extra hard outside of practice with a "do whatever it takes type of attitude". Truth is, I didn't know what it took until I started doing my own research and testing on my own body.

I typically beat my competition by outworking them, but I used extreme dieting methods. I learned these methods from my high school coaches. Just like I was learning from other people, you will know by learning from me. I will be your mentor because I already went through all the BS with low-carb this, take this supplement, "oh dude, you need to bulk you're looking kind of small," "oh dude, you need to cut, its summertime," take this pill or needle and you'll get huge and cut man. I have seen it and I've been through all of it, except for anabolic steroids. I am here to tell you that there is a better and more efficient way. Yes, that's right you heard me. There is another way and it is quite simple!

Up until the age of 22, I was doing it all wrong. Like most of you, I was the guy digging my head in bodybuilding magazines and buying all these supplements to try and bulk up or shred down. If you are a teenager reading this, then you can strongly relate. This didn't work, so I turned to professional bodybuilders for advice. Just like you reading this book, right now, I was reading bodybuilding books. Finally, I learned some facts and things started to click! The only downside was every book I turned to was based off of steroid use so I had no way of knowing whether the programs were legitimate or not.

So I tried, and I tried, and I experimented.

At the age of 22, I was going through my master's program and broke up with my girlfriend at the time. That was when I decided to take my training to the next level. I wanted to compete. So I read anything and everything I could get my hands on. I came up with a solid workout plan, and I started to count calories. I really wanted to figure this bodybuilding stuff out. Furthermore, I turned to a local bodybuilder in the area named who also coached other people up into their shows. I went into the "pose room". The pose room was a dark and gloomy room underneath an old school iron gym. That was where I met the guy. He was surprised at how much muscle considering I trained naturally. I was 230lbs, I benched over 350lbs, and squatted over 450lbs. There was only one problem; I was bulky. I had no definition because I ate so much and used numerous types of supplements to try and get big. I wanted to look like the guys in the fitness magazines, but I didn't know how to keep my size and still look shredded.

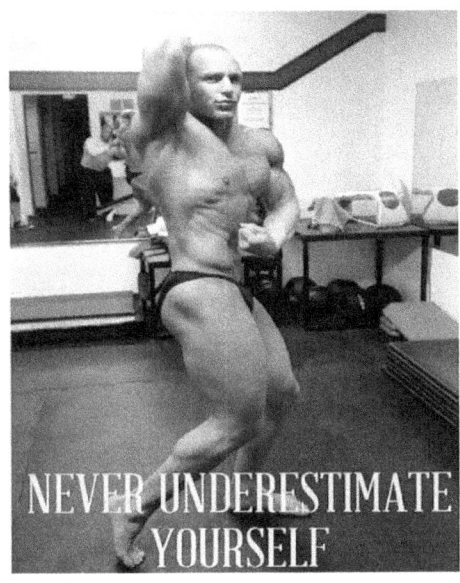

-The Pose Room. This is where I met with my coach every Sunday.

We met every Sunday on my lunch break and I would pose and switch up my dieting methods. Most of the time, we would just cut more calories. I was big and strong just like the pre-roid bodybuilders. These were bodybuilders I looked up to, like Steve Reeves and Reg Park. These guys were my idols. They were the bodybuilding kings before the 70's when steroids changed the scope of bodybuilding. I trained like them and ate like them. I kept my lifts heavy and ate carbs for the first time in my life while training and dieting. Yes, I ate carbs, over 350 grams while cutting! I didn't really listen to my coach all that much because he wanted to cut my carbs out right away and I knew that if I cut my carbs I would lose all of my mass really quick. My coach was very helpful with posing and telling me whether or not to lean out or to develop this muscle group further. He was a judge for NPC division, but he took steroids. He asked me to take them with him and I turned him down because I knew I stood for something different. This was difficult, being coached by someone who used anabolic steroids and I knew that I couldn't train like him or eat like him because I was natural, so I engineered my own training and dieting style by educating myself.

For my first show, I placed second. Excuse my language but I was pissed. I had worked so hard and came in second. I had 30lbs on the guy who beat me too. That day I learned what bodybuilding was all about. Bodybuilding is all about perception. Because I held my carbs throughout the show, I also held my glycogen storage; therefore, I wasn't as cut as the guy who beat me. He also posed a little bit better in the main show and the pose down, I will give him that.

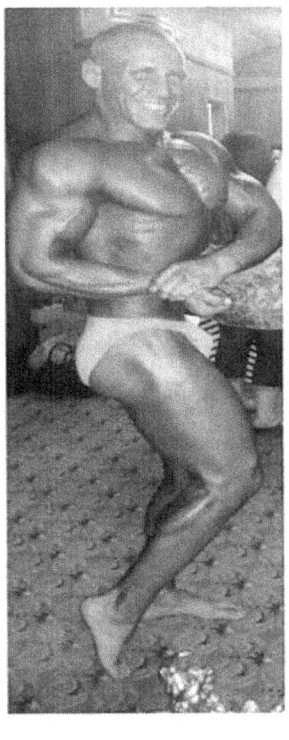

-My first bodybuilding completion. Notice the fullness.

If you guessed I went on to do a second competition, you are right. I had 6 months until my next competition and I had to move. I had to come up with a new strategy and a new game plan, so I called the main judge in my previous show. He said I needed to lean out more to gain more saturation (to show more muscle). I did more cardio and I reduced my calories even more. I lifted the same. Yes, I didn't change my work out a bit. I wanted to challenge the typical status que of changing your workout so I could get more shredded. I worked out the same five days a week, did more cardio, dieted harder and got shredded. I'm not talking the typical, "oh man, I can see your muscles now" shredded. I am talking fitness model shredded.

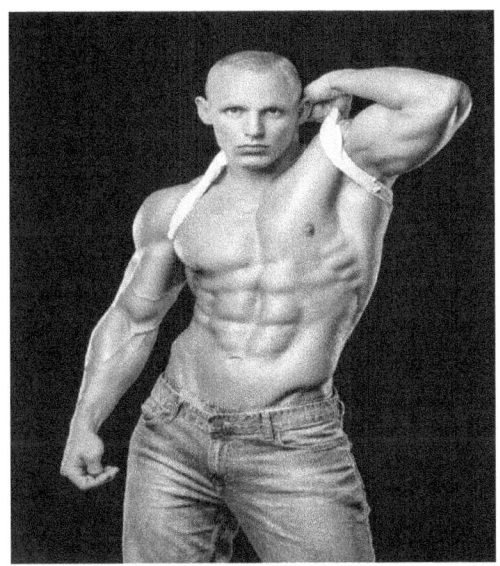

-A photo taken from a photoshoot a week before the Pro-Natural show in Las Vegas.

5

I felt so confident in myself, I asked the hottest girl in town out who turned out to be a model. My world had suddenly changed from just being an average Joe to muscle model status, having a hot girlfriend, and I drove a Suzuki Samurai. Yeah, she didn't care about my car one bit. What she liked, was the confidence I had. This confidence carried on to my job and I was a top producer my first year at the job. It was like I was living a movie just by making some simple changes. I figured it out and I would like to guide you through the process of how to improve your health and reach you goals.

I am not writing this book for profits like many industries; instead, I am trying to educate people on how they can achieve the body of their dreams NATURALLY by receiving the correct information and following the correct steps. I want to save YOU time, money, years of hard work, frustration, and years on your life. Just like any industry, education can only be one stage of growth and development. You must go out and apply the principles to receive results you've always dreamed of. If you read this book and apply the principles, your life will change drastically.

If you are lacking self-confidence, if you are overweight or underweight, if you spend countless hours in the gym and see very little results, it's not your fault. You heard me; it's not your fault! There is so much BS information and supplements out there that people don't know what to believe anymore. If this is you, it's okay, I've been there. I was the fat kid with no self-confidence. I couldn't get a date and I was screwed. I would try this supplement or this workout plan to try to become big and shredded. If you decided to change yourself, you decided to purchase, put your head down, read, and apply you will be on journey to a much better you and maybe even a competitive you.

The information given in this book applies to all age groups. From 12-years old, to years over 50, this information will apply to you. Age is just a number. Literally, I know natural guys that are in their 50's and look better than when they were in their early 30's.

Part I

Chapter 1: How to Read this Book

You're probably thinking, "Okay man, I know how to read". I totally understand, a lot of people do nowadays, but this book is a little different. This book was made with just enough of the most valuable information to where you can take it to the gym without having to lug around a huge dictionary. There are also QR-Codes placed within this book. You will need a smartphone and you will need to download a QR code reader in the app store of your smartphone. The QR code will look something like this:

They will be placed throughout this book; mostly for video links to make sure you are doing your exercises properly and to make sure that you make every rep count. Can I ask you for a favor? I ask that you be a sponge and absorb all of the knowledge that you can from this book. The goal here is not to keep your head in this book forever, but the goal is that you educate yourself, use this as a reference, and jot down your results of every set and loss or gain in the back of this book.

One Question, Are You Ready?

Chapter 2: The Secret to Success in Health & Fitness

Let me let you in on a little secret, there is no such thing as a perfect physique. Just be the best you can be. I just want to say I helped you on your journey. ~Your Author

-Goals and Vision

If you are lost, you have asked people on what to do or how to work out, it's okay. I remember going up to one of my best friend's father and asking him what to eat for bodybuilding because the dude was huge and a trained ex-NFL athlete! Yeah, he was on steroids, but he did introduce me to one of my favorite super foods, a sweet potato. I will start by asking, are you confused? Do you know whether to eat dairy, bread, ice cream, fruits, or even meat? I'm sure you have heard people say, "If you want to get cut and shredded, you shouldn't eat any dairy". You may have heard this one, "Don't eat after 6pm or you'll get fatter than a beach whale!" That one is my favorite. Last but not least, I'm sure you have heard the saying, "eat all your carbs in the morning, and don't eat any carbs for your last 3 meals or don't eat any carbs for three months to shred up for that big summer event". Ah, let me tell you, not eating carbs sucks! I'm sure most everyone can agree with me there. Your irritable, light headed, you have no energy, and you can't think or function properly.

There is so much information out there with the emergence of fad diets and the evolvement of anabolic drugs since the 70's. A fad diet is a phase diet, meaning the diet is popular at first and it will phase out after a couple of years. Some fad diets that you have probably heard of are the Atkins, Paleo (not bad just too much fat), raw food, South Beach, alkaline, blood type, the five bite, even the werewolf diet. Yeah, some guy came up with a werewolf diet, can you believe that? Eat these foods and you'll turn into a werewolf and you'll get all the chicks just like Twilight. Pretty fancy huh? Again, there is so much "fluff" out there. When you see someone promoting these types of diets, ask them, "How much weight have you lost?", "How much muscle have you gained?", "Hey man, you look like you're going to pass out, how's that diet going?" The truth is, these methods don't work and if you've tried these diets and failed miserably, it's okay. Don't worry, I'm here to tell you are in good hands.

Lies and Misconceptions

You may be asking yourself, "Why haven't I ever heard of a simple step plan to getting the body I always dreamed of?" because the supplement companies and fast food ventures want you to keep buying their product or food. You see girls and guys in the gym constantly drinking their protein shakes? Yeah, I can tell you first hand that they are conformed by the supplement industries and they consume way too much protein. Too much protein will make you fat. You don't pee out extra protein because protein is a calorie. You may even see the huge powerlifter in the gym who eats burgers and fries for a post workout but they can't ever seem to see any type of muscle definition. They are working their tails off just to stay in some sort of decent shape. Who wants to live the type of lifestyle in being in a constant struggle to keep weight off? It's no fun.

Another reason why you have never heard of a program like this is because bodybuilders have huge egos and are some of the most selfish people on the planet. I know because I was one of them. They will literally hoard their information and knowledge just to make themselves look better. Most are on anabolic drugs and believe that taking harmful drugs and eating burgers, fries, and pizza is the only way to become big and strong. Then when it comes time to cut, they take other anabolic cutting agents to strip away all the junk they ate. We call these people "juice heads".

Chapter Three: The Real Science Behind It All

Do you remember in science class when your teacher told you, "The trees need sunlight, water, and nutrients to grow?" I won't go into biology because I know that learning biology isn't your goal, but your body works the same way as the trees and plants. What? Yes, it's the same concept. We all need water to survive, the sunlight is your workout (resistance and cardio), and nutrients come from the food you digest. It can't be that simple right? News flash, it is! What? The multi-billion-dollar supplement industry wants you to believe it's a lot more complicated, but it's really not.

I'm sure you have pondered on this- What is a calorie? Or what is a protein? Or what is a carbohydrate? Or what is a fat? Is there good fat or bad fat? How much protein do I need? Are all carbs bad? We must understand these concepts in order to develop the healthiest looking tree or human body possible. I think you can understand my analogy usage. I will explain how we will do this in later sections. Yes, there will be some boring information but guess what? It will be worth it. You've tried and failed numerous times over and over again. So you have to ask yourself, what do you have to lose? Will you know more than most of your friends that will stay on the same diet fad or even no diet? I can tell you after reading this next section, you will become more knowledgeable than most, especially the guys trying to sell you on fitness dream that will never come true at your nearby corporate gym.

What is a calorie?

A calorie is a unit measurement of energy potential. Even coal has calories. Yeah, like the coal used to run ships and trains back in the days. For this book, we will be only focusing on the human body form of calories. These calorie types include proteins, carbohydrates, fats, and alcohol. Let me ask you this, have you ever woke up, went to work, and skipped breakfast. You probably feel tired and drained throughout the day right? This is your body sign that you are lacking on energy. Your body may even go into starvation mode and shut off all fat burning in the process. I will go into this under the section labeled metabolism.

Protein

A protein is a calorie source that builds and repairs muscle cells when broken down. A protein can be broken down further broken down into amino acids. There are a total of 27 amino acids and amino acids are the building blocks of protein.

Carbohydrate

A carbohydrate is a form of energy that is made up of 3 main atoms being carbon, hydrogen, and oxygen which are all the same. No, not all carbohydrates are created equal.

Fat

Fat is the oil found in animal or plant based products that are used in cooking. There are certain fats that are better for you than others.

Alcohol

In fitness terms, alcohol is also a source of energy. Alcohol is considered an empty source of calories because it has very little nutritional value. Consuming alcohol diminishes testosterone and reduces the amount your body burns for energy.

Nutrient

A nutrient is a needed source to fuel the body to grow.

Metabolism

Your metabolism is key to fat burning and muscle growth. Your metabolism will break down molecules from food to release energy, which is then used to fuel the cells in the body and to create more complex molecules used for building new cells; hence, the faster your metabolism the more energy (food) you need. Metabolism is necessary for life, and it is how the body creates and maintains the

Anabolism

Anabolism is a metabolic procedure where energy is used to make more complex substances (such as tissue) from simpler ones.

Catabolism

Catabolism is where the body basically eats itself through the production of energy by breaking down complex molecules (such as muscle or fat) into simpler ones. This is what happens when people generally "cut".

Macronutrients

Macronutrients are your main drivers of caloric sources being protein, carbohydrates, and fats. You may have heard the phrase, "If it fits your macros" (IFYM) eat it. This is a method used to count calories. Some people abuse this method to eat like crap and they will still lose weight. Yes, you can eat junk food and lose weight. There have been studies, such as the nutritionist Mark D. Haub who ate Twinkies and who lost 27 lbs. in 10 weeks[23]. I don't advise you doing this because of health reasons but it can be done. Remember, we are in this for the long haul. So try to stay away from junk! Although this method is abused I strongly believe in this method. In fact, this is the only method for one to truly know where he or she is at when leaning out or gaining muscle.

Micronutrients

Micronutrients are extremely important to health. Micronutrients provide the body with nutrients. These are your vitamins, amino acids, fiber, and minerals. You can meet all the macronutrient goals you want, but if you are not getting the proper micronutrients you will feel bogged down, achy, tired, and you might even lose your hair. That's why you see a lot of bald bodybuilders. I won't go into detail about each one, but just know if you are not eating a nutrient dense diet (vegetables, fruits, etc.) you will most definitely need a multi-vitamin supplement. Oops I said it, yeah I said supplement.

Supplement

A dietary supplement is used to provide nutrients that may otherwise not be consumed in sufficient quantities through a regular diet. Yep, that is a definition of a dietary supplement. If you don't believe me, look it up. News flash, you don't need a whole lot of supplements. In fact, you won't need any if you have a balanced diet.

Now that I have you amazed, with some simple scientific terms. We will go into further details regarding nutrition.

Chapter Four: Nutritional Breakdown

If you want a better future, it's not going to happen automatically. You have to make it happen by will, work ethic, and knowing the facts ~ Your Author

Okay so now that you have a glimpse of what certain terms mean to get you to a much better you, we will go into a little in depth concepts. Don't worry and don't be scared, these concepts will only help educate you.

Diet

A diet is the amount of food or drink a person consumes. A diet can be regulated for one to lose weight or gain weight by restricting or adding on calories.

Healthy

This is a big debatable word for most people, but when it comes down to it, it's really quite simple. Healthiness means that one's body is in great physical and mental condition. Health is measured by one's strength, endurance, energy, and immune system.

FRUCTOSE

Fructose is a sugar found in many plant sources like honey, fruits, flowers, and root vegetables.

SUCROSE

Sucrose is the kind of sugar most commonly called "table sugar" like the sugar you may drink in your pre-workout and not even know it. Sucrose is made up of glucose and fructose. Sucrose can be artificially produced but it can also come from fruit sources. You will want to stay away from all table sugar are maltodextrin sources as they are imperative to your overall health.

GLYCOGEN

This is the big concern to everyone. This is the big scoop on the low carbohydrate diet being. Glycogen is a substance stored in the liver and muscles in the form of glycogen that can be broken back down into glucose if needed for energy. The body stores glucose in the liver and muscles in the form of glycogen, which can be broken back down into glucose when energy is needed. You know that bogged down feeling you get after an intense workout? That's a sign that your glycogen levels are low.

BLOOD SUGAR

Blood sugar levels are defined as the amount of glucose in your blood. Glucose is carried in throughout and delivered to blood cells. This process breaks down glucose and that energy can be used or stored for later use.

SIMPLE CARBOHYDRATE (AKA the Bad Carbohydrate)

A simple carbohydrate is a carbohydrate where the body can break down quickly into glucose. This carbohydrate is widely used for a quick burst of energy. Examples of simple carbohydrates are the fructose found in fruit, the lactose found in dairy, and sucrose, maltodextrin, dextrin and sports drinks or energy bars. Pretty much anything that tastes sweet is a simple carbohydrate.

COMPLEX CARBOHYDRATE (AKA the Good Carbohydrate)

A complex carbohydrate is a carbohydrate that is made up of a chain of simple carbohydrates linked together. Because of its structure, it takes the body longer to break it down into glucose. Examples of complex carbohydrates are the sugars found in grains, legumes, and vegetables.

STARCH

Starch is a complex carbohydrate that is found naturally in many fruits and vegetables, and it is sometimes used as a food additive. Many particular foods high in starch break down into glucose quickly, like a simple carbohydrate would. Vegetables that are high in starch include corn, peas, parsnips, potatoes, pumpkin, squash, zucchini and yams.

HORMONE

A hormone is a chemical produced in the body that controls and regulates the activity in specific organs. In males the dominate muscle producing hormone is testosterone. In females, the dominant hormone is estrogen.

INSULIN

Insulin is a hormone that is manufactured by the body in the pancreas. Insulin is released into the blood when you eat food. It causes muscles, organs, and fat tissue to absorb nutrients from food, which are also released into the blood, and either used or stored as body fat. Furthermore, Insulin is very important for your metabolism and utilization of energy.

GLYCEMIC INDEX

The glycemic index (GI) is a scale the measures the effects of carbohydrates sources on one's blood sugar level. Complex carbohydrates are broken down and release glucose into the blood slowly (good carbs) are low on the GI index. Simple carbohydrates that break down and release glucose into the blood quickly (bad carbs) are high on the GI index. 55 and below on the GI index is considered low, and anything above 70 is considered high. Glucose is measured as 100 on the GI index. This is very important and you may view a scale just by searching for a GI index online. So you may get the gist, Complex carbs break down slower, which makes less likely to add fat storage because you will hopefully be burning your energy throughout the day. Simple carbs are a bam and wham type of carb if you are not doing sprints or a high enduring sport or refueling from a vigorous activity you are adding a large amount of stored glucose to your body (fat) which will have to be burned off later. Refer to the chart in the tools section for more information.

PROCESSED

Processed food is made using chemicals or machines to preserve it. Preservation methods remove most of the nutrients that the foods naturally contain. In some circumstances, the chemicals used to preserve the food are toxic to the body. Even your protein bars can be harmful. What? Yes, they are processed.

GRAIN

Grains are a seed of different types of grasses, and are used in many types of foods.

WHOLE GRAIN

Foods that contain grains that have not had parts removed are called whole-grain foods. Examples of whole grain foods may include brown rice, whole grain breads, and whole grain pastas.

WHEAT

Wheat is a plant that makes grain. Hence, if you are eating whole wheat bread, you are eating ground up wheat plant and grain.

WHITE BREAD

White bread is a processed bread that is made from wheat flour and has grains removed and has been bleached so it bakes easily with greater longevity. This bread is purely human engineered. The process of making this bread removes most of the nutrients from grains, making the bread into a simpler form of carbohydrate. Stay away from this "stuff".

FIBER

Fiber is a type of carbohydrate that the body cannot digest. Fiber assists the body's regulation of sugar. Fiber is found in many types of foods, including fruits, vegetables, legumes, nuts, and grains. Fiber is important when keeping a level glucose level which is very important in muscle building. So, eat fiber filled foods!

FATTY ACIDS

Fatty acids are the molecules that make up fat cells. Some fatty acids are needed to build parts of cells and tissues in the body. Fatty acids contain more than twice as many calories per gram as carbohydrates and proteins do. Fatty acids are mainly used to store energy in fat cells.

ESSENTIAL FATTY ACIDS

Essential fatty acids are fats that cannot be synthesized by the body; therefore, the body must receive these fats from its diet. There are two essential fatty acids are linoleic (omega-6) and alpha-linolenic (omega-3). Linoleic acids can be obtained by eating peanuts, salmon, tuna and more. Alpha-linolenic acids can be obtained through walnuts, flaxseed oil, canola oil, soybean oil, red meats and dairy products.

CHOLESTROL

Cholesterol is a waxy substance that is found in two sources: your body and food. Cholesterol is necessary for survival and is used in building the cells and vital hormones in the body, as well as for other important functions. All the cholesterol you need is produced through your liver and circulates it through your blood. Too much cholesterol in the blood, however, increases the risk of heart attack, stroke, and other disease. [1]

Cholesterol comes from foods such as meat, fish, eggs, butter, cheese, and whole milk.

Cholesterol is not found in foods made from plants. You should have no more than a 100g of daily and no more than 50g if you have heart problems.

LDL (BAD) CHOLESEROL

LDL cholesterol is considered the "bad" cholesterol because it is a main driver to plaque which clogs arteries and makes them less flexibles. LDL cholesterol is one of the leading causes of a blood clot, heart attack, or stroke. My advice is to avoid saturated fats and oils, such as butter, bacon drippings, lard, palm oil, and coconut oil. Wait are all LDL cholesterol fatty foods bad. No, use olive or canola oil when cooking if needed and eat oatmeal, kidney beans, apples, pears, barley and prunes. Research also shows that people who increase their soluble fiber (oat, seeds, lentils, some fruits and vegetables) intake by 5 to 10 grams daily have up to a 5 percent drop in LDL.[8]

HDL (GOOD) CHOLESTEROL

HDL cholesterol is considered the "good" cholesterol because it helps remove the bad cholesterol from your arteries and prevents the death factors up above. HDL foods include avocado, fatty fish (ex. Salmon), flaxseed, nuts, and soy. Seriously, this is like magic and will improve blood and mineral flow; hence, more muscle growth.

BODY COMPOSITION

Your body is composed of two types of mass being body fat and fat-free mass. Body composition is the proportion of fat and fat-free mass in the body. A healthy body composition contains a higher proportion of fat free mass (muscles, organs, tissues) and a lower proportion of body fat.

BMI

BMI is known as a person's measurement of body mass index. It is based off of a person's height and weight. This method is not very accurate because it does not take into account of muscle mass or body fat.

BODY FAT PERCENTAGE (BFP)

Body fat percentage is an actual measurement of body fat that your body contains. If your body fat is 20%, that means 20% of your body is fat. Don't freak out! Your body needs a certain percentage of body fat to survive and the rest is just fat. There are different methods of measuring body fat and some methods are more accurate than others. The skin caliber or an electronic censoring machine is the most popular methods used because they are the cheapest and the most time efficient. Don't stress too much on body fat just worry about how your feel and how you look in the mirror.

REP

A rep is one complete motion of a specific exercise.

SET

A set is a group of continuous repetitions.

Boom! You got through the tuff stuff. You learned so much, right? You know have an AA in life fitness definitions. Congrats! Now, I will mail you a nice shiny diploma. I'm totally kidding, but take these terms and store them in your memory bank, like a sponge, because they will be vital for the rest of your life.

Chapter Five: Myths & BS

"Hey man, I got this new rabbit horn extract buy it and you will get huge" or "Take this pill, with an extract from an ancient ocean front property in Idaho and you will lose 20 lbs. in a week" -Your Local Bioscience Expert

-Do more cardio to get a lean muscular looking body

This is my favorite one. Well you can if you want to be a skinny twig. The more muscle you have on your body composition, the more calories your body will need to fuel this muscle; hence, fat loss. Guess what? You'll have to eat either way you might as well eat to fuel muscle mass instead of fat mass.

-I can lose body fat in my problem areas

Wrong. You cannot control where you lose body fat. If you are in a caloric deficit, you will lose body fat and you cannot control where you lose it from. Men tend to store body fat in their stomach areas while women tend to store body fat in their legs or thigh area. Everyone is different though, it just depends on last spot where your body disposes of fat. Personally, my thighs are where I store the most body fat.

-Man, I can't do it just because my genetics suck

After you become educated on the concepts in this book, get up, and go workout. Genetics is a lame excuse for an, "I can't". Yes, some people do have better genetics than others when it comes down to digesting different types of macronutrients, especially energy sources. I remember asking myself, "why can all my friends down cheeseburgers and tacos (loaded with fats, carbs, and calories) and I can barely eat a sandwich and gain body fat." It's because my body just processes sources of calories differently. I decide to stick to something and I made changes to engineer my body and I figured it out. I figured my body out, I figured how calories work, and I stuck to my workout while everyone else was making excuses.

-More sets and more reps equal more muscle

Not necessarily. Your body will be broken down in the aftermath of a challenging workout. You will need to heal. If you're a beginner, you shouldn't do over 16 sets because it's just too much. For an advanced person training, you shouldn't do any more than I remember back when I read the Arnold bodybuilding book and followed his program. My body was sore, I could barely even move and I had to repeat the same workout every other day. Don't get me wrong Arnold is one of my bodybuilding idols, but he took anabolic steroids. This meant he could heal a lot faster, than a natural person trying to obtain a great physique. I worked my butt off and I wasn't getting results. I was in the gym for two and a half hours a day. Sounds familiar? Get your head out of the magazine workouts and diets. A workout shouldn't last any longer than an hour and a half with cardio.

-I need surgery to get rid of my cellulite

Cellulite is nothing more than fat underneath your skin. Get rid of the fat and you get rid of the fat. Plain and simple.

-I need a coach or trainer to make my body look "good"

I have been in this spot before and totally messed everything up because a coach or a trainer doesn't know your pains, workout history, or your stamina. Only you know yourself best. All I can say is believe in yourself! One of my ex-girlfriends I had just didn't believe in her own techniques and paid over $800 a month to a "guru" body coach when she was a kinesiology graduate! Yeah, she looked great, but just didn't believe in herself enough. I fell into this trap after getting feeling a strong connection with coaches and receiving results. I was coached by two of world's top natural bodybuilders. I won't say any names, but one is the best in the Professional Natural Bodybuilding Association and the other is the best in the International Federation of Physique Athletes. I wanted to learn from the best first hand and I did. I can tell you I learned a lot from them, but what I got from both of them was to believe in yourself.

-Almond milk, Soymilk, and Rice Milk is just as good as milk

Although almond milk is marketed as a having more calcium than milk, the calcium is not the same. Almond milk's calcium source is an additive from ground up sea shells. Because your body requires vitamin D to absorb calcium, almond milk and soymilk companies usually partner calcium fortification with an extra dose of vitamin D. Since cow's milk is already calcium rich, only extra vitamin D is added during food processing. After fortification, cow, soy, almond and rice milk are approximately equivalent in calcium and vitamin D concentrations, delivering about 30% of your daily need for calcium and 25% to 45% of vitamin D in each serving.[5]

-Salt is "bad" for you

Salt is a necessary nutrient and without salt, we would all die. Seriously, sodium deficiency is a medical condition called hyponatremia. It affects about 3 million U.S. citizens per year.[20] Have you ever been to the zoo or the horse stalls? If you have, you usually see salt blocks in their cages or stalls. Animals, just like humans need sodium to conduct life or their nerve and muscle cells will not work properly. Sea salt should be your only form of salt you eat.

A lot of the time bodybuilders will like to load and deplete their sodium levels in order to "shred up" for a contest. This is a really tricky method and you must count every gram to make it work. It can be done, but it's not advised and it's not healthy.

-If I cut my carbs, I will get shredded

Yes, you can get shredded from cutting carbs but most the time your protein and fat caloric intake raises because you are hungry. When this happens, you are still consuming the same number of calories, so you will not lose fat. Cutting carbohydrate calories while keeping protein intake and fat intake around the same margin is the quickest way to lose fat. You totally deplete your glycogen stores (fat stores). But while cutting carbs, you will lose a considerable amount of muscle. This is bad. Remember we want to keep as much muscle as possible. So what's the right answer you ask? We want to diet down while keeping a balanced macronutrient profile. Studies show that when proteins are more likely to be digested when digested with a carbohydrate source, the body functions more efficiently.

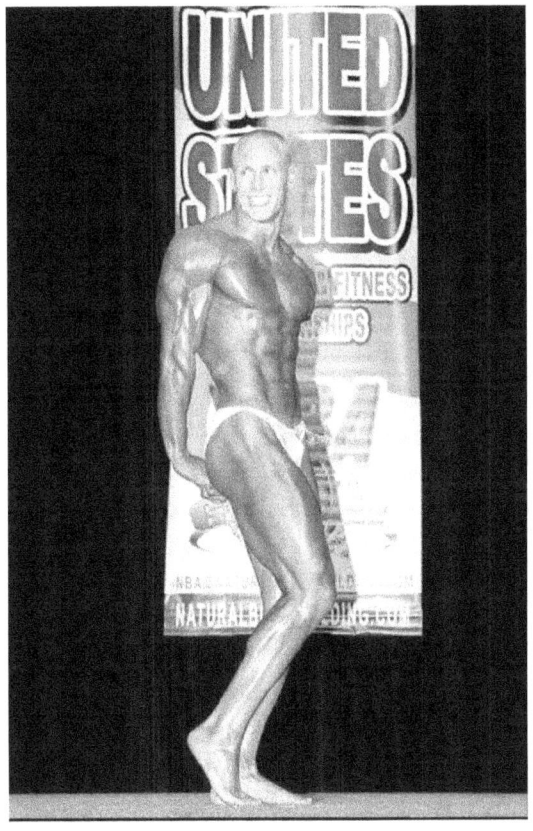

-After cutting carbs down to under 100 grams while consuming a low amount of a fat intake under 60g for several weeks. I was also doing 250 min of cardio a week for several weeks. I did whatever I took to win this show. I lost over 5lbs of muscle while trying to drop my body fat to an extreme level. I didn't like the way I looked but the judges liked it. I DO

NOT RECOMMED THIS!!

-If I work hard enough I will get there

Hard work is great and I love your determination. Every athlete must have this mindset, but they must be educated behind their trade. Knowing how the body works and reacts to different food and nutrient sources is crucial. You know why a Ferrari requires 91 octane? It requires that high of fuel octane because it is made to perform at peak conditions (quick & fast). This will be the same case for your body. Therefore, if you want to have a prize physique and feel good it is a package deal. Well you can give it 20% and just workout, but who wants to just give a 20% effort.

-I have to take steroids to get big or ripped

No you don't. You will be surprised where your natural genetic potential can take you if you put the correct time and effort in and out of the gym. Plus, who wants to be unhealthy like that anyhow?

-I have to eat 6-8 meals a day to have a great body

Incorrect. I've done 8 meals a day for a year straight and it is a lot of work. Your body will optimize your carb/fat/protein sources more efficiently if you decide to eat five to seven meals a day, but it is not necessary. Five to six meals a day is a good enough spread to where you can fit in all of your macronutrients needed while speeding up your metabolism. Remember Steve Reeves? He only consumed 3 large meals a day which equated to about 1,800-1,900 calories. His diet consisted of a 35% protein, 40% carbohydrate, 25% fat ratio and he was Hercules. Yeah, he was the very first Hercules that trained only 3 times a week. You can eat 3 meals a day and have a great looking physique because it's been proven.

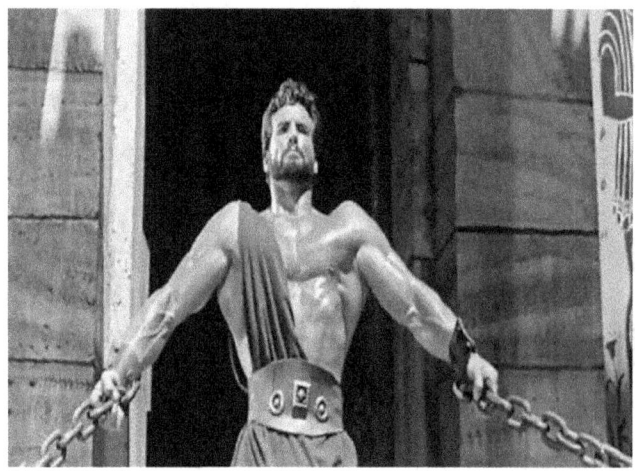

1947 Mr. America Steve Reeves-Bodybuilder, Hercules, Actor, Philanthropist

-A competition diet is only chicken and broccoli

No, this is an old school bodybuilding method. If you do this, you will wind up nutrient deficient because you will not get enough sources of food. This is about the same method when high carb, low-fat, low-protein came about in the 1980's.

-If I do lots of ab workouts, I will get abs

Well, you already have abs and they are just hidden underneath body fat. Your abs should start to show at about 12% body-fat (males) and 17% (females) if you work them correctly. You can make your abdominal muscles bigger by training them, which will make them protrude more over your belly fat. I do not recommend a bunch of transverse movements (side-bends) because they will build up your transverse abdominals and make your waist bigger. If you want a slim waist, stay on top of your nutrition and training. Remember building the body you want is all about health and proportions.

-I NEED pre-workout before I go to the gym

No, this is what the supplement industry wants you to believe. Have you ever heard of Pavlov's Dog experiment of classical conditioning? Pavlov fed the dog several times and the dog salivated. Pavlov then went on to ring a bell and the dog did not salivate. So Pavlov went on to ring the bell while feeding the dog food, and the dog salivated. Guess what? Pavlov rung the bell with no food and the dog salivated. This is the same case to your attachment to pre-workout before your workout. You work out because you want to look good and be healthy. Okay, then you think I have to have this pre-workout because it going to help me out and get me there quicker. Yeah, pre-workout may improve your focus and may give you a better "pump". I will warn you that most preworkouts these days have too much caffeine (bad for your heart in large doses) and laboratory made stimulants that give you a high but they will mess with your hormones (like bedroom performance hormones). So what do you take before you exercise if you need a little boost? Green Tea, because it is all-natural, loaded with antioxidants, and has just enough caffeine to get you up and going.

-That guy is big he must be super strong

Not all big guys are strong. In fact, most bodybuilders these days are quite weak. They use a method of training called hypertrophy to where they pump up the blood and nutrients into one muscle group. This is where you get that "Swollen" feeling, but you have to be in the gym for hours. I know because I have done it. Power lifters on the other hand aim for strength and care very little about being shredded or aesthetics. These are the big and strong guys eating over 6,000-calories a day. So how do you get the best of both worlds staying lean, big, and strong while maximizing time and effort? That's what you will learn from this book.

Part II- The Fundamentals of Exercise

"The journey of a thousand miles must begin with a single step." -Lao Tzu

Okay, you made it through part one. Give yourself a pat on the back and do some push-ups because you are so pumped for part II. I am totally kidding, but if you want to do push-ups more power to you. Anyhow, in part II we will cover more of the mental factors behind fitness and reaching your goals and full potential.

Chapter Six: Success Lies in You

"Training is like life, you get your ups and downs, but if you think about your problems hard enough and logically enough, you'll either solve them or reach a compromise." -Reg Park

Now that you are reading this book, you will become educated on how to reach YOUR goals. Furthermore, there will be little to no one to put the blame on. No more blaming your fitness/health goals on fad diet or a workout program. Like so many people, when the New Year hits, they become super motivated and drop off. Then you never see that person in the gym again until next year and they are even heavier than before. There is a valid reason behind this. It's because they don't know what they are doing.

If I went to the gym and worked my tail off for 2 months, ate decent, and really wanted to see results but didn't. I also would want to quit. It's kind of like going to work and not getting paid. It's not fun and it is a waste of time. These are usually the people on the treadmill for hours or the people on machines. Let me tell you something about machines fitness equipment. It was invented to sale gym memberships to people that don't know what they are doing. They figured that people would hop on this machine and follow the diagram and see minimal result. Just enough to spark consumers' interest and think they are benefiting themselves. The truth is, you will see some results, but it only lasts for so long.

You, me, and everyone else needs something that works. We literally thrive off of detailed plans. We say, "Okay, he or she received results doing this. Why can't I?"

If you have worked out hard in the past then quit, did you ever ask yourself why you quit? I can guarantee you it's because you worked so hard and never seen results, or maybe it was because you didn't see results fast enough. You started to come up with excuses left and right why you shouldn't work or eat healthy. Then you start to feel sorry for yourself or maybe you get pissed off. Let me tell you, I have been there. I tried the mediocre fitness lifestyle and it was a complete disaster. I can assure you that you have taken a step in the right direction. Hopefully, this will motivate you.

-Sphere of Influence

Have you ever felt like you lacked motivation? Whether it's getting fit, eating healthy, or asking that pretty girl out on a date, you may be letting those around you hold you back.

It doesn't matter if you have the golden ticket; if you are in a bad environment, you will eat the chocolate. They say you are the average of 5 people you spend the most time with. In fact, there is a widely known theory known that backs this principle up named the social bonding theory. The social bonding theory states that people have attachments to families, commitments to their schools or employment, involvement in activities, and they believe that these things are of importance. [6]

-Change your environment & change your mindset

You may have to change your sphere of influence to change your mindset. In order to grow mentally, physically, and or spiritually, you must have a growth mindset. You may have to lose some of your friends that don't have this type of mentality and or mindset to become a better you. These people that don't have this type of mindset will hold you back if you let them. For example, when I decided to start bodybuilding, I only hung around those that were also into bodybuilding and fitness. One of my good friends which I will mention later on, decided to make the switch too to competing in physique and he is also a pro athlete. So if you want to get fit and be healthy, start socializing with those that have the same goal in mind.

-Bad Habits

Tobacco won't affect my performance or make me look worse. I hear so many people say this over and over or you may even see the tuff guy coming out of the gym to grab a cigarette for his post workout. I was a victim of tobacco usage once because I hung around those that also chewed tobacco (sphere of influence). I still worked out hard as hell and ate all my protein, but I couldn't ever get my physique to change from puffy to lean. I would push my body so hard while running that I would start gagging.

I became the case of my own classical conditioning experiment because I made it an effort to run until I made myself either puke or gag. It was then I thought I had worked hard enough. I thought I had run hard enough to complete my cardio session. I thought, if I only push myself harder and harder, I will get there and I will get the lean, big physique I always dreamed of even though I am chewing Tobacco and drinking alcohol. No, this wasn't the case at all. Once I decided to change my sphere of influence (I was doing rodeo at the time), I was able to quit the nicotine and alcohol consumption fairly easy. I kept lifting and running, and for the first time in my life I got down to 14% body fat and had a full set of abs. I still didn't have much of a clue on what I was doing but I pushed myself 6 days a week for about three hours a day and had a full set of abs.

-But I'm Scared to go to the Gym

Personal motivation is one thing, but being afraid to go to the gym is another. I hear this phrase so many times, "what do you have to be afraid of?" Being afraid to go to the gym is unrealistic; it is more of a lack of motivation.

Here are some strong motivators that may apply to you: I want to lift weights so I can excel at a certain sport, I want to run on treadmills so I can eventually climb a mountain, and I want to take a yoga class to calm my mind and ease my anxiety. These are legitimate motivational reasons for someone to attend the gym.

-The One Thing

If you really want to get fit, be healthy, and have a nice looking body you will have to focus your energy. You have the most energy and willpower in the morning. The more you exert your willpower in the morning to complete a project for school or send emails, the more likely you are to be worn out by the end of the day. Therefore, you will be less likely to go to the gym and exercise. Check out Gerry Keller's the one thing for more information on this theory. If you want to focus on your health, I suggest doing your most important task in the morning. The morning is when you have the most will power.

-All in All

The objective here is to find motivation. Motivation can come from an external source or even an internal source. External motivation will come from those around you. Do your friends want more in life, do they want to push themselves in their career/business, and do they want to be healthy? Internal motivation will come from you and only you. Remember when I said my grandpa passed away from obesity. That is my main motivation. As of now, I would like you to write down your motivation on a piece of paper and hang it somewhere where you see it every day. Examples of this can be your fridge, mirror, or up above your desk. If you see it, you can believe it. I bought a poster of Steve Reeves and hung it up on my wall, practiced his classic poses, and had the focus in my workouts just like he did. If it is a look you want, then find someone you want to look like. If you want to make money, you find someone who makes a lot of money and you ask them, "Can you teach me to make money".

-Your Mind Is Your Most Powerful Muscle

The Body Achieves What the Mind Believes ~Your Author

Your mind controls everything. Seriously, you are what you believe. Just like you are what you eat. I believed that I could go pro in natural bodybuilding and I did it within three shows. I believed that I could get an MBA and I did it. I believe that I can help other people achieve their goals and I will do it! If you don't believe you can't do it, you won't. Do you ever ask yourself, I wonder how he or she got to where they are at? It's because they got educated on the right information and they believed. Jim Carrey visualized and believed he could become famous and make 10 million dollars in 3 years.

He did it on the set of Dumb and Dumber. Don't believe me, check this out https://youtu.be/-CbAcNDuEyA. Once Arnold retired from bodybuilding, he believed he could be the next Hollywood box-office star. Everyone turned him away and said there was no way. His vision and belief was so powerful he made it come true. There was Terminator I, II, III, and so on.

If you can get one thing from this book, it is I want you to believe in yourself and the process. You will discover great treasures when you act and you practice like it is impossible to fail.

Now that I have your attention, I ask that you write down where you're at and where you would like to be.

Current Weight:_____   Goal Weight:_____

Chapter Seven: Muscle Growth (AKA Gains)

All right, now were getting into some interesting facts. Here it is, muscle growth is defined as $X+Y-E=R^2$. I'm totally kidding, but this is what all the "Bro Science" bodybuilders and supplement companies want you to believe. I was a victim to this for about five years of my life. The keys to muscle growth are really quite simple and they have been for a century now. It is the same steps that all the pre-roid bodybuilder used to do. Building muscle is all about completing the right tasks. So what are the right tasks you ask? It's all about pushing your muscles until failure and fueling enough with the right nutrients.

Now, there are several ways to do this being strength, hypertrophy, and endurance. I don't want to confuse you because this is a step-by-step process but just know that strength requires (6 reps or less & 3+ min of rest), hypertrophy requires (8-12 reps & 6090 sec rest), and endurance entails (12+ reps & 30 sec rest). Hypertrophy and endurance workouts are great workouts depending on your goals, but for this book we will be focusing on a strength workout that will build muscle and shred body fat. This workout program will be a similar method as to what Vince Gironda, George Eiferman, John Grimek, Leroy Colbert, Reg Park, Steve Stanko, Jack Delinger, Steve Reeves and many more have used to build prize winning pre-roid era natural physiques.

Our bodies are still functioning the same way they used to back before the use of steroids and unhealthy fitness practices so why wouldn't the pre-roid methods still work today? The cool thing is- they still do! Bodybuilding has evolved into something unhealthy in today's age and the average lifespan of a bodybuilder of today's age is relatively short due to heart failure.

Reg Park (Late 50's)	John Grimek (30's-40's)	Vince Gironda (Late 40's)

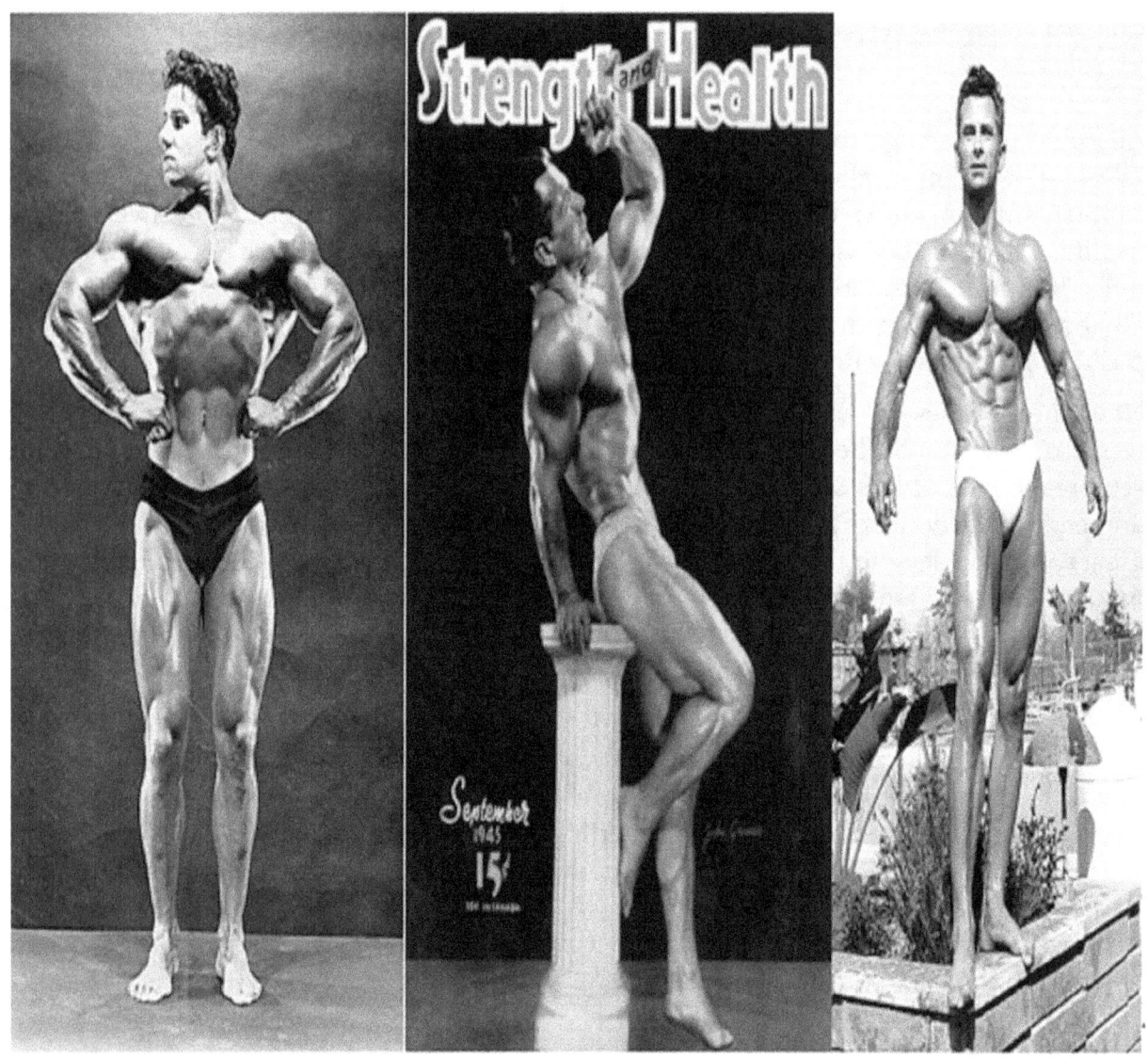

-Building for Strength

Now-a-days, bodybuilding is all about volume. Volume training was a method developed during the 70's (steroid era), to build mass fast doing 10 sets of 10 reps. "Do 25 reps with a 45 sec rest period and you will blow up", said one of the steroid using bodybuilding coaches I had. I'll admit volume training does pump the blood into your muscles and it hurts pretty bad, but it doesn't build you up or lean you out. When you come out of the gym after doing a volume training session (5 sets of 12+ reps) you will feel drained; furthermore, your muscles will flatten out. If you want to be lean and healthy while build a balanced physique like the bodybuilders above, keep reading.

Let's face it; Arnold Schwarzenegger changed the bodybuilding industries in the 70's. Before he changed the industry, he had to learn from someone. He looked up to and learned from Reg Park (https://youtu.be/oK8baGoSoR8). This is how Arnold built his base for his mass. He then went on to a high volume training method that is being used nowadays. These are the typical training styles you see in the muscle magazines. How did the bodybuilders train before high volume and anabolic steroids? They trained for strength. They lifted heavy and they grew. I used the same method to go from 210 to 230 in 3 months while maintaining abs. I grew dense muscle and I had tons of energy that kept my workouts fun and exciting. I was in the gym for no more than 3-4 days a week and no more than an hour and a half in the gym. No training splits of 5-6 days a week in the gym.

So what's the compound lifting method and what does it consist of? How do we train like Hercules (Reg Park and Steve Reeves were both Hercules)? It's really simple and is built off of compound lifts. Compound lifts are multi-joint exercises; that means you use more than one joint to perform the lift. These lifts include deadlifts, Romanian deadlifts, squats, bench press, incline press, pullups, bent over rows, standing shoulder press, dips, and barbell curls. These workouts give you the most bangs for your buck. You burn the most calories and build the most muscle doing these exercises.

Think about it. Your whole life, you are either pushing, pulling, squatting, or lunging. You want to be the strongest and most balanced in these four motions. Pushing exercises consist of a bench press, incline bench press, standing shoulder press, or a dip. Think of these motions as pushing a door open. Pulling exercises consist of pullups, curls, Romanian deadlifts, bent over rows. Think of these motions as pulling a door open. Squatting motions are basically squats and deadlifts. Think of these exercises as squatting down on a chair. A lunging motion can be condensed to a forward lunge. This motion is used for a sudden thrust forward. Unlike a useless motion, such as a shoulder shrug, these motions will keep you flexible, strong, and give you proper bone strengthening for the rest of your life. Ask yourself this, do you want to be the old person being pushed around by your grandkid in a walker? Or do you want to be the old person chasing after your grandkid on his bicycle? Do your compound exercises.

-Full Body Routine

Yes, you will be doing a full body routine. A full body routine provides the body with blood circulation in all major muscle groups, adequate rest, muscle balance, lesser chance of injury and great results naturally. This program works well because you can balance it with your work balance life being Monday, Wednesday, and Friday. The sweet thing about it is you only have to be in the gym for 3 days a week and you can do your cardio while going on a hike, swimming, bicycle riding, a brisk walk, basketball you name it. No more gym rat status or gym burnouts because there is more to life than being in the gym 24/7 trying to perfect something that will never be perfected.

Chapter Eight: Get with the Program

Fortunately, there is a solution, and it's not performing multiple sets of whatever cable Kegel exercise is being pushed as "The Answer." Just a little hard, smart, basic work." - Jim Wendler

TRAINING CALENDAR

Novice Routine

Workout		Set | Rep	Details
Hyperextension		3 | 10	**Rest:** Take 2 min rest between sets.
Bench Press		4 | 5	
Deadlifts		4 | 5	
Barbell Squat		4 | 5	**Duration:** 3 Days a Week for a 3-month Duration.
Seated Calf Raises	Day 1	3 | 6	
	Day 2	3 | 15	**Workout Length:** Will take you about 60 minutes without chit chatting in the gym
	Day 3	3 | 6	
Leg Lifts & Stability Ball Crunches		3 compound sets until Failure	

Intermediate Routine

Workout	Set | Rep	Details
Hyperextension	3 | 10	**Rest:** Take 2 min rest between sets.
Barbell Squat	5 | 5	
Bench press	5 | 5	
Standing Barbell Press	5 | 5	**Duration:** 3 Days a Week for a 3-month Duration.
Upright Row	5 | 5	
Deadlift	5 | 5	**Workout Length:** Will take you about 70 minutes without chit chatting in the gym.
Standing Calf Raise	3 | 25	
Leg Raises & Reverse Crunches	3 compound sets until Failure	

Herculean Routine

Workout	Set | Rep	Details
Upright Rows	3 | 8-12	
Bench Press	3 | 8-12	**Rest:** 60 sec rest between sets & 2 min between each workout.
Bent Over Barbell Row	3 | 8-12	
Dumbbell Laterals	3 | 8-12	
Incline press	3 | 8-12	**Duration:** 3 Days a Week for a 3-9 month duration.
Dips	3 | 8-12	
Barbell Curls	3 | 8-12	
Standing Dumbbell Curls	3 | 8-12	**Workout Length:** Will take you an average of 90 minutes without chit chatting in the gym
Dumbbell Pullovers	3 | 8-12	
Squats	3 | 8-12	
Deadlifts	3 | 8-12	
Hyperextensions	2 | 8-12	

Calf Extensions *Leg Press Machine*	3 | 15	
Leg Lifts & Stability Ball Crunches	3 compound sets until Failure	

Deserter Routine

Workout	Set | Rep	Details
Hyperextension	3 | 10	
Front Squat	3 | 8	
Squat	4 | 6	**Rest:** Take 2 min rest between sets.
Romanian Deadlift	3 | 8	
Standing Barbell Press	5 | 8	**Duration:** 3 Days a Week for a 3-month Duration.
Standing Lateral Raises	4 | 10	
Bench Press	4 | 5	**Workout Length:** Will take an average of 105 minutes to complete & you won't want to chit chat.
Incline Barbell Press	4 | 8	
Pull-up (use assist/weight if needed)	5 | 8	
Barbell Row	3 | 8	Give it all you got.
Barbell Curl	4 | 8	
Dips	4 | 8	

Standing Barbell Calf Raise	3 | 25	
Standing Calf Raise	3 | 25	
Leg Raises & Reverse Crunches	3 compound sets until Failure	

Hyperextensions	2 | 8-12		Dips	4 | 8	
Calf Extensions / Leg Press Machine	3 | 15		Standing Barbell Calf Raise	3 | 25	
			Standing Calf Raise	3 | 25	
Leg Lifts & Stability Ball Crunches	3 compound sets until Failure		Leg Raises & Reverse Crunches	3 compound sets until Failure	

Chapter Nine: Keys to Training

Do you ever see guys in the gym doing reps as fast as they can or doing heavy weight with horrible form? I can tell you first hand, that their ego is too big. They will end up hurting themselves or they won't make any progress and they will quit working out for a year or so. So what are the secrets to training? The secrets to training are intensity, tempo, focus, positivism, overloading, and progression.

Workout intensity can be defined as how much energy is expended when exercising. Your intensity can vary based upon your rest times and overloading. Steve Reeves and Reg Park's workouts were high intensity because their short rest periods and focus on overloading each muscle group. Workout focus is defined as feeling and making every rep count by thinking nothing else besides muscle contraction. Remember your mind is the most powerful muscle in the body.

Workout tempo is defined as the pace that a rep is performed. Lowering the weight is called the eccentric motion. Focusing on an eccentric motion can be 1.75 times more effective than solely focusing on the concentric motion.[18] Believe it or not, more muscle is built off of the eccentric motion because you have more control. The midpoint is where you will hold the weight for 1-3 seconds before pressing. This pausing motion is called an isometric motion.

After I read Steve Reeves book, I would hold the weight in the downward motion for a

3 second pause and I built a lot of muscle and strength in a short amount of time. Everyone eventually thought I was on steroids because of how well this system works. If you are lacking legs, I strongly recommend this method. The pressing up, pulling down, or curling upward motion is the concentric motion. When using this style of workout tempo, you increase the time under tension of each muscle group worked; therefore, you will increase your growth.

The positivism in a workout is directly related to workout overload and progression. Being positive and telling yourself you can move and control the weight will make the difference between a great workout and a poor one. Workout overload is defined as the continuous process of increasing demands of each muscle group worked in order to grow and progress. In order to become bigger and stronger, you must believe and continually lift more to make your muscles grow. If you don't, your muscles won't become bigger, nor stronger. In other words; if you don't use it, you will lose it.

Chapter Ten: Cardio

What about the other 5 days of the week? What do I do? This is what I thought at first and the same with all of my clients. "Well, I have to stay active or I have to lift if I don't I will lose all of my GAINS", says who? This is a total misconception. Another wide misconception these days is, cardio is evil or for skinny people. Not true, cardio is very important to heart, vascular, circulatory blood flow, longevity, and overall vital health. What muscle supplies nutrients by pumping blood into your muscles? If you answered your heart, you are right. The American Heart Association recommends you have complete at least 150 minutes of moderate activity (can talk, but not sing) or 75 minutes of vigorous activity (hard to talk) or a combination of both.

It is true that too much cardio can hinder muscle growth if you are not consuming enough calories. Take Michal Phelps for an example, the Olympic gold medalist swimmer, he eats 12,000 calories a day. He eats a lot, but he does a lot of cardio. Steve Reeves ate 3 meals a day for a grand total of 1,900 calories. What is different about these two athletes? Physiques and the amounts of cardio they do. Steve Reeves was active outside his training days in the gym and loved to power walk for health.

So what's the answer and what's the plan? Well, your cardio needs are based off three different factors being, your caloric intake, fat mass, and fitness goals. If you are trying to lose fat mass, I recommend building muscle, eating a caloric deficit (less than what you currently eat), and doing no more than 5 cardio sessions. If you are trying to gain muscle mass, I recommend doing cardio only on your off days (days not training) at but staying very active. So no more than 90 minutes of cardio a week.

What is the best cardio and when is the best time to do cardio? Let's start by defining cardio. Cardio is short term for cardiovascular exercise and is any exercise that raises your heart rate. Cardio can be playing your favorite sport, walking, running, or using equipment at your gym. There are two types of "labeled" cardio being LISS and HITT. LISS stands for low intensity steady state (60-80%) of your max heart rate. Generally, your max heart rate is 220 minus your age, unless you are very athletic. LISS is an awesome method of cardio if you are trying to build muscle since your heart rate will stay low during your cardio session, you will primarily be burning body fat for fuel. Once your heart rate gets too elevated and into the 80-90% of levels, you primarily burn glucose. Of course, you are burning calories during cardiovascular training, but your body is fueling itself from different sources. Keeping your heart rate at a moderate level for 30 minutes ensures that your body will burn fat as a primary source for fuel instead of muscle.

HIIT cardio is a method of cardio that stands for High Intensity Interval Training. This is a relatively new method of cardiovascular exercise that incorporates an 80-90% target heart rate for a short burst of time followed by a LISS recovery period. For example, walking for 2 min or light jog followed by a 30 sec sprint repeated for 25 minutes. Research shows that HIIT leads to similar and in some cases better improvements of heart stroke and metabolism in shorter periods of time then LISS. Here is the secret, use a method of both so you do not get bored with your workouts.

The best time to do your cardio for fat loss is in the morning on an empty stomach (fasted), directly after a training session, or in the evening after dinner. In these methods of cardio timing, your body will be completely depleted of glycogen. It is not advisable to do cardio directly before resistance training because your body needs the calories you just ate to fuel your workout for muscle growth. Furthermore, if you train in the morning do your cardio at night or on your off days and vice versa.

Chapter Eleven: Stretching

Believe it or not, stretching should only be performed after your workout session. If you stretch beforehand, you are more likely to create tears in your muscles, which could lead to larger tears when training. While exercising, your muscles tend to shorten. Stretching after your workout helps lengthen your muscles for greater adaptability, posture, and flexibility. Each stretch should be held for 20-30 seconds. I won't go into much detail about stretching and the different methods. If you feel as if you must stretch before your workout, try warming up with a lighter weight instead of stretching.

Part III: Exercises & Muscle Groups

When completing your exercise routine, your exercise form should be at the upmost importance. Your form will make the difference between gaining muscle and strength without breaking an arm or leg. We must first understand how to do the exercises to perfect form, so let take a look. In this chapter, I will explain the basics of all compound lifts that you will be enduring in your new lifelong exercise routine.

Before I can show you the explanations of the exercises, you must get familiar with the main muscle groups. Use this image table below for a reference guide when looking for muscle certain muscle groups.

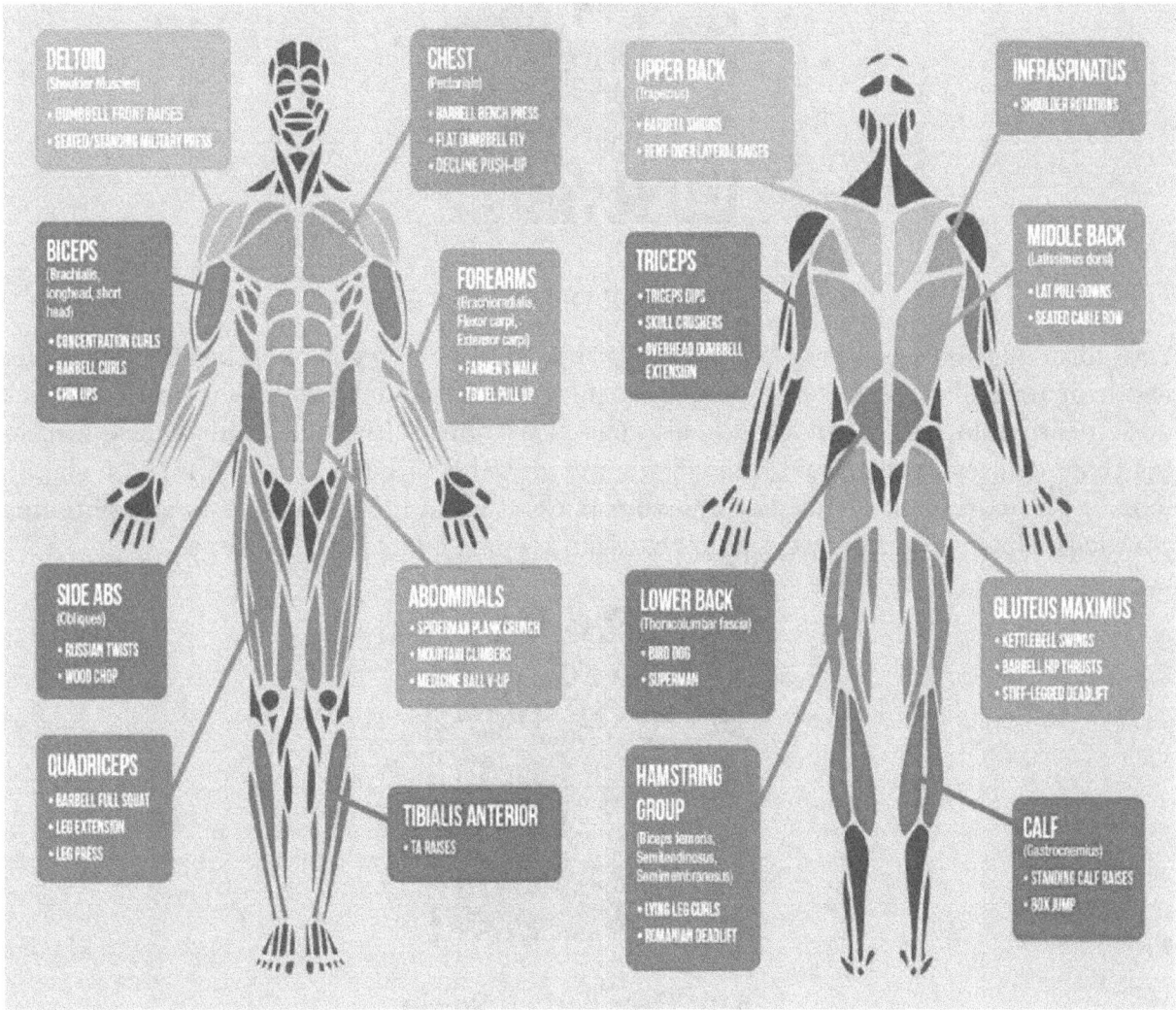

-Hyperextension

This exercise is a lower back isolative movement (non-compound) that will assist in strengthening your lower back for compound movements such as a squat and deadlift. This exercise also is a nice stretch for your erector spinae (lower back). Beginners do not need additional weight for this exercise. You can make this exercise more difficult by adding body torque. Body torque is putting more tension on the desired muscle group by using your arms or legs as levers. Think of this concept as a pipe wrench on a bolt that won't come loose. If you get a bigger wrench, it is easier to break the bolt loose because you are adding additional pressure. This is how some exercises work. With a hyperextension, start by placing your arms across your chest on a hyperextension bench. Complete a set by isolating and pausing for 3-seconds when you're fully extended. If this isn't enough resistance, move your arms to the back of your head, then lock out in front. Finally, if this isn't enough pressure you can repeat this process by adding weight.

-Barbell Deadlifts

Your form on this exercise will be extremely important. Your feet should be about shoulder width apart and your knees should be bent. You should have a step-up or a block underneath your feet for an additional range of motion. With your hands a little further out than your legs, you should reach down and grab the barbell. At this point, you should look like a figure four. While keeping your back straight, lift the weight by straightening your legs. Slowly lower the weight down, while keeping control. Then, repeat.

-Bent Over Barbell Rows

With your feet shoulder width apart, your thumbs in an "in-ward" position, grab the barbell a little wider than your knees. Your knees should bent while maintaining a straight back. Pull the barbell upright to your chest, pause, and slowly lower the barbell back down. Your core should remain tight and contracted. Focus on achieving a full range of motion on every rep.

-Pull Up

Pull ups with a wide grip, are the number one exercise for developing a wide lateral spread. If you desire a skinny waist and a wide back look, you do not want to skip this workout. To complete a pull up, grab the pull up bar with your arms slightly wider than shoulder width. Pull upright until your chin fully clears the bar. Slowly, lower back down maintaining time under tension. You should maintain an arched lower back while completing this exercise.

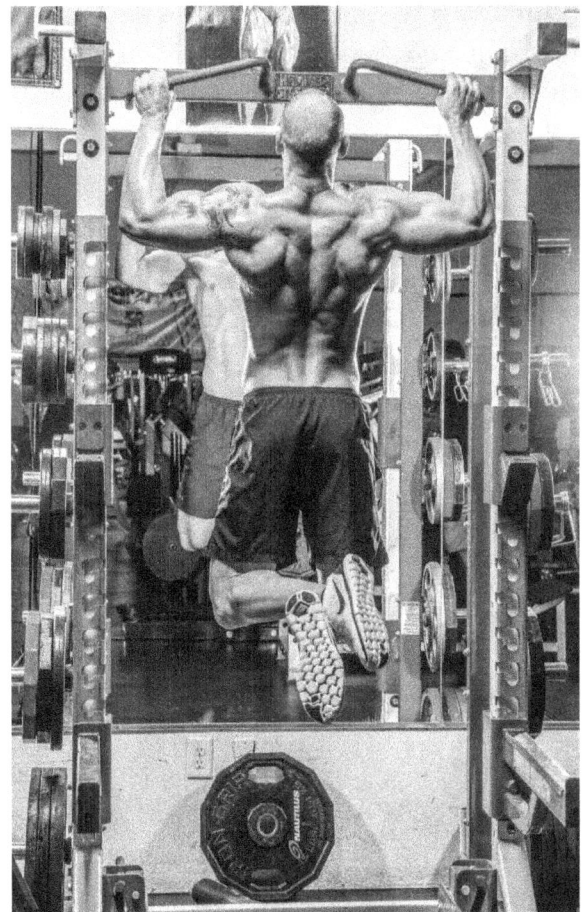

-Lat Pull Down

Sit on the lat pull down machine and take a wide grip on the overhead pully bar. With your thumbs in an "in-ward" position, arch your back, and pull the bar down, to the V in your neck. Make sure to keep your elbows forward. Pause. Slowly let the bar come up and repeat.

-Barbell Bench Press

When you think of working out, you think of bench press. When someone asks you, "Hey man, how much do you lift?" You also think of the bench press. The bench press is performed with your back and your feet up on the bench. Grip the barbell at about 18 inches wider than your shoulders; slowly lower the barbell down to your nipples, pause, and press the barbell upward directly over your chest. Repeat.

-Incline Barbell Press

This is an upper chest focused workout. Implementing an incline barbell press into your workout routine makes your chest appear much fuller. Lie on an incline bench, while grasping the barbell slightly wider than shoulder width apart. With your wrists straight, lower the barbell until it touches your upper chest. Make sure to keep your elbows pulled back. You do not want to complete an incline press while keeping the bar drifted on the lower chest. This will take the tension off the upper chest and places it on your lower chest and front deltoids.

-Dumbbell Pullover

A dumbbell pullover is a compound movement that uses the upper chest, lats, and serratus (wings). To complete a dumbbell pullover, lie on an exercise bench, while keeping your feet up on the bench and your head off up off bench. Place your palms on the underpart of the plates of the dumbbell and hold the dumbbell over your head with both hands. Take a deep breath and expand your rib cage while lowering the dumbbell behind your head. Keep your elbows slightly bent while pulling the dumbbell up over your head until you pull it over your lower chest. Focus and Repeat.

-Squat

A squat is the number one compound movement for developing the legs and glutes. To do a squat, you should be underneath the squat rack, while hold the barbell on your traps. Keep the bar balanced by holding the bar with a wide grip. Slowly lower the weight while keeping you head up. Keep your knees pointed directly out in front of you, toes straight, back tight, glutes (butt) tight, and keep your shins perpendicular to the floor. Lower the weight until your quads and glutes are parallel to the floor. Pause and then come back up. The squat takes some time to master, if you are a beginner, it is extremely important to be in full control in this workout. If you feel like your posture is off in squat exercise, lower the weight and try again.

-Front Squats

This workout activates your thighs. Grab the barbell with a shoulder-width apart grip. Clean and pull the barbell up onto your deltoids. You may either support the bar with your wrist and deltoids, by holding your elbows forward or you may cross your arms while keeping your elbows up to keep the bar resting on your deltoids. Lower the bar while keeping your lower back and core straight and tight. Squat all the way down until you reach parallel. Pause and come back up. Repeat.

-Leg Press

If performed correctly, this workout activates your thighs. It is a much more isolative movement than a squat because it does not require as much balance. In this exercise you will sit in a leg press machine with your lower back pressed up against the back pad. If you have lower back pain, slightly lift your butt up off the seat. Place your feet on the lower part of the platform about hip width apart. With your hands behind your thighs (control), lower the weight until your thighs touch your ribcage. Return to the starting position without locking your knees. Repeat.

-Romanian Dead Lift

This workout activates your hamstrings, glutes, and back. For all of you ladies reading this, this is a workout you don't want to skip. To perform a Romanian dead lift, keep your grip about shoulder width apart, place your feet up under a block or step-up, and grab the barbell with an overhand grip just outside your thighs. Keep your knees slightly bent and arms straight. Pull the bar up while activating you hamstrings and glutes. While pulling you should be thinking in a mind to muscle state. Make sure to keep your lower back arched and core tight to prevent injury. Lower the bar bar or weights until they are one inch off the floor. Repeat.

-Barbell Lunge

This workout is a burner or a burn-out workout. Meaning, it should be performed last. When performed correctly, the lunge will activate your thighs and glutes. To perform a lunge, hold the barbell on your traps, just as you would on a squat, step forward with your right leg while keeping your core tight. Bend your knee until your thigh is parallel to the floor while keeping your left leg back and straight as possible. To activate your glutes on this exercise, keep your right shin perpendicular to the floor while looking up. Return to an upright position, pause, and repeat.

-Standing Barbell Press

With your feet about a foot apart, grab the barbell with your hands about shoulderwidth apart. Clean the barbell up onto your clavicle bone just above your chest. Press the barbell straight up while keeping your core tight. Slowly, lower the weight down and repeat. Make sure to achieve a full range of motion on this exercise.

-Standing Dumbbell Lateral Raise

Lateral raises are the primary exercise for building your side deltoids. If you desire a small waist wide shoulder look, this is a workout that you do not want to skip. Start by keeping your feet shoulder width apart and keeping the dumbbells out in front of your thighs. Keep your elbows slightly bent while raising the dumbbells laterally while twisting your palms to a frontal position. Remember, the longer the lever the better. Pause once your shoulders have reached the same height as your wrist and dumbbells. Slowly lower the dumbbells and repeat.

-Standing Bent-Over Lateral Raise

This exercise will activate the rear deltoid muscles. With your feet a little wider than shoulder width apart, grab your pair of dumbbells. Keep your knees and arm slightly bent. With your back bent and head up, raise the dumbbells smoothly out to your sides. When the weights are parallel to the floor, pause. Slowly lower the weight down and repeat.

-Dips

This exercise should be completed with a parallel bar. In this exercise, you will want to keep your elbows near your sides while bending your arms and lowering your boy as far as you can. Press yourself up, using your triceps. While maintaining control, slowly lower yourself down. Repeat. Note, you may place your feet behind your torso (activates more of the lower chest) but if you want to activate more of your triceps and core, keep your feet out   in   front   of   your   torso.

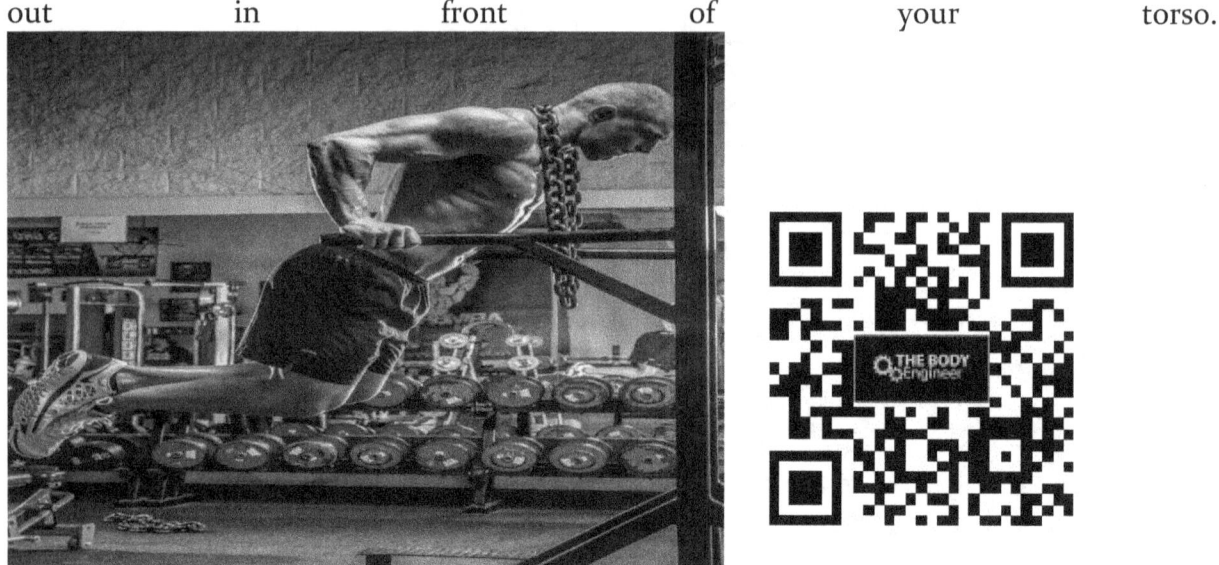

-Standing Barbell Curls

With your feet about shoulder-width apart and a barbell held in a 'palms up' position. Curl the weight up to your chest and pause. Slowly lower the weight. It is important to keep your elbows by your side and back in line with your waist. Do not swing in this exercise. If you have to swing in this exercise, you will need to lower the weight.

-Standing Alternate Barbell Curl

With a pair of dumbbells in your hands, stand with your feet a little narrower than shoulder-width apart. Curl one dumbbell up to your shoulder with your elbow back and near your side. Slowly lower the dumbbell while curling the other. Repeat. Note- if you feel like you're up for an extra challenge, you can flex your triceps when your dumbbell is down near your side.

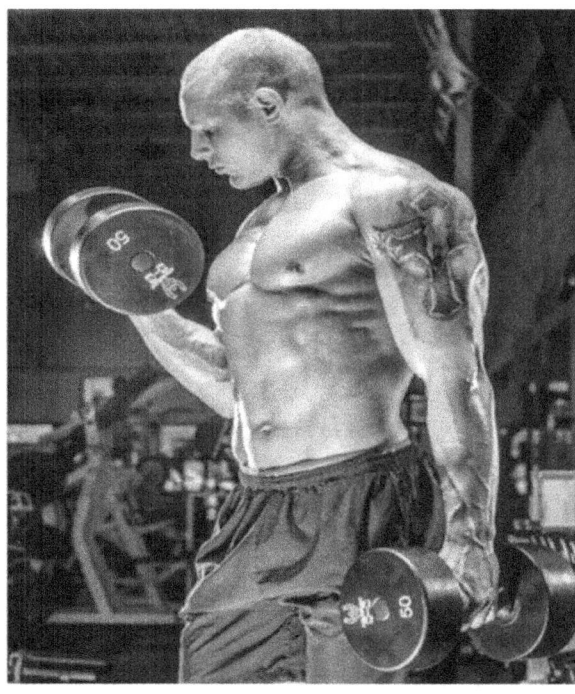

-Seated Calf Raises

With your knees tucked in, sit on a seated calf machine. Your feet should be about a foot apart and you should place your feet to where you can press the weight up off of the front of the ball of your feet. Slowly lower the weight down and press up as far as you can, using the ball of your foot. Pause, slowly lower back down and repeat.

-Calf Raises (Smith Machine and Step-up)

When you need to work out your calf muscles, you usually go to a standing calf machine or a seated, but what if there are none around? A smith machine calf raise is your answer. With the smith bar up, place a step-up or a block underneath the smith barbell. With your toes up on the step-up, rest the bar on your rear deltoids just as you would in a squat. Twist the bar, press up as far as you can using the ball of your feet, pause, and slowly lower the weight back down. Feel the burn, and repeat.

-Leg Raises

Using a vertical bench, place your forearms on the armrest. Grip the handles while keeping your back up off the backboard. Raise your legs outward while keeping your legs locked. Pause in the upward position, slowly lower your legs, and repeat.

-Leg Lifts

This exercise will be very similar to leg raises. Using a vertical bench, place your forearms on the armrest. Grip the handles while keeping your back up off the backboard.

Lift your knees up near your chest and slowly lower your legs back down. Repeat.

-Stability Ball Crunches

Sit on a stability ball and slowly walk your feet out in front of you. Your lower back should be near the midpoint of the ball. Stretch, excel and crunch up simultaneously, pause up top for 3 seconds, slowly lower back down, and repeat. Note- this is a great exercise to build balance and your core. Make sure you get a full range of motion and use your arms as levers just as you would in a hyperextension. Don't be scared. If you fall backwards on your face, you can always get back up.

-Reverse Crunches

Lye back down on a bench. While grasping the bench with your palms, lift your legs up to your knees then push your legs up as high as you can. Slowly, come back down with your legs, in the same orderly fashion and repeat.

Do I Need a Weight Belt?

Unless you are maxing out (one-rep) or you just want to look cool like those guys you see wearing a weight belt for every single exercise then no you do not need a weight belt. In fact, a weight belt will actually hurt you more than it will help you. When wearing a support belt, you are taking pressure off your lower back and core while completing a compound lift. In turn, your core will actually get weaker than stronger. If you continue to wear a weight belt or support belt when completing an exercise, you will always need the added support.

Difference Abdominal Training

Do you notice that there are only 2 different sets of abdominal exercises? In each and every compound exercise, your core (abdominal) is strengthened; hence, there is very little need for core exercises. Your abdominals will show when you're at a low body-fat percentage. So why are there abdominal exercises listed in each program? These abdominal exercises are longitudinal abdominal exercises. Long are those that are used to trim your waist, not make it bigger.

If you would like a large waist, then you can load up the ab machine with weight and do 8 reps of 5 sets

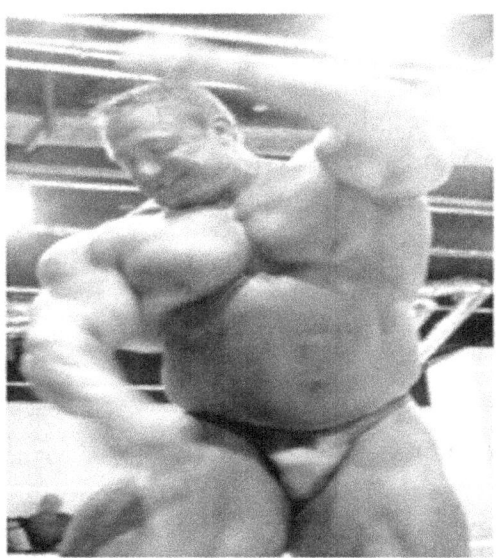

like the bodybuilders in today's age.

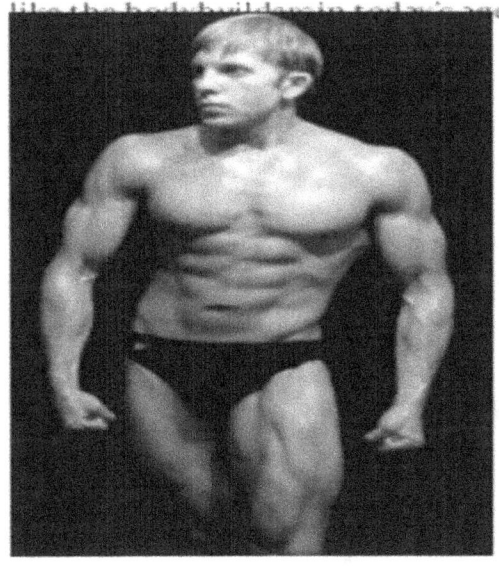

Vs

If you would like a trimmed and small waist, to make all of your other body parts POP follow the exercises in this program.

Gender Differences and Training

I know you may be thinking, "But I'm a woman, I can do these workouts". There are very little differences between males and females when training. I'll explain these minor differences in below:

1. Gender has little to do with metabolism and performance. These factors can be explained by size and body composition.

2. The main gender difference has to deal with the difference in sex hormones and Type-1 fiber types.

3. Women are better equipped at handling both carbs and fat (calories disposed for energy or storage) due to a difference in muscle tissue; hence, women tend to have better metabolic health.

4. All of these differences make women better metabolically suited for... just about everything related to health and performance except for short, intense bursts of activity that rely on glycolytic capacity.

On average, men have 2/3 more muscle mass then women, mostly in the upper body area. Although, there are some very strong women, men tend to be stronger than women because men tend to carry more muscle mass. Sorry ladies. Both men and women produce the hormone called estrogen, but women tend to produce more. Estrogen plays a major role in woman's metabolic health and insulin sensitivity. I'm sure that there are men reading this, thinking maybe estrogen is a good thing. Well, it is to a certain extent. You will want to keep your estrogen levels normal with endurance. Endurance trained men are more likely to have increased muscle sensitivity to estrogen which improves your muscle glucose uptake and metabolic health. Woman tend to have more Type-1 fibers which have the ability to provide more blood to the muscle in order to provide a greater oxygen, glucose (carb), and fatty acid (fat) absorption[22]. The only place where men have the advantage is glycolytic capacity (breakdown of glucose) and explosive performance (short aerobic burst).

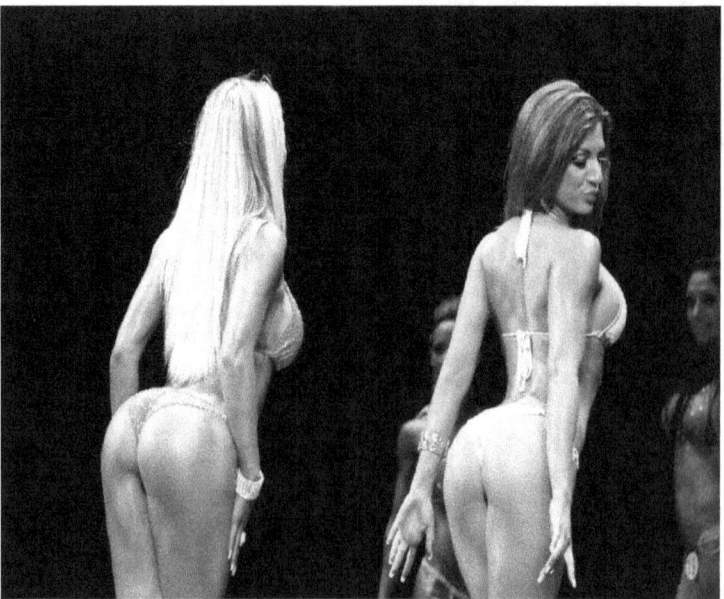

Another thing I must mention, if you're a woman and you lift weights, you will not get huge and look like a man. This is may be a perceptional issue, but most of the woman that look like men lifting weights are using steroids. Lifting weights and being active is actually really healthy for woman and may be extremely attractive to some men. If you find yourself being able to beat up your boyfriend, good for you.

Part IV: You Cannot Out Train a Bad Diet

Second by second you lose the opportunity to become the person you want to be. Take charge of your life. ~
Greg Plitt

Some people say it's 70% some people say it's 80%, but I say nutrition is 100% of your results. Your nutrition is fuel to the fire. It's a compass while your sailboat in the ocean. Think about this for a moment, how are you able to start a campfire? You need wood, a match or a lighter, and kindle (gasoline or lighter fluid) to start a fire. How do we keep a campfire lit? We have to keep throwing wood on it correct? If the fire burns out, you are going to freeze. Your body works in the same manner. If you don't fuel your fire, you will never get it started or you will lose it all. Just so you know, I am speaking in terms of muscle here. To sum this up, you must eat to build muscle.

What the heck do I eat? This is the number one question of all time. There are a couple of different methods to this. Method one, is eating "healthy" foods. I'm not talking the food that is claimed to be healthy at your local fast food joint because it is processed and full of preservatives. Just look at the back of a label and actually look what food producers put in some foods. I am talking about whole foods vegetables, fruit, whole grains, eggs, steak, poultry, fish, nuts, and dairy. With this approach, it is very simple you just pick certain foods, eat until you feel full, eat them every day, and change your portions based on feeling. You either eat more or less depending on weight loss or weight gain. Another approach to eating is a new approach called MACRO or IFYM (if it fits your macros) dieting. With this approach, you calculate your macronutrients (protein, carbs, and fats) for your daily intake and you have a lot of variety in your foods. This approach is very flexible and it will allow you to go out and eat with your buddies, eat processed foods, or your family just by plugging your foods into an application on your mobile phone. This method does have its pitfalls though. Macro dieting requires a lot of thought process, takes a lot of time out your day, and most of the time you end up lacking important micronutrients. Last but not least, is a micronutrient and macronutrient approach. This is the method that I recommend because I have personally achieved great results. With this approach you eat whole foods and count your macronutrients. This allows balance the balance you need to be social while maintaining a great physique.

How Much Protein do I Need?

Just like you, I have read on all the bodybuilding forms saying, "Whatever you do, don't drop your protein". I tried this method for many years and I got "Big" but I was always poufy looking. I wasn't that healthy either and then I started educating myself. Let me tell you, there is no such thing as too much protein. I have been trained by some of the best natural body builders in the world today and none of which suggest a huge amount of protein. There are numerus studies out there with different protein requirements form healthy day to day living to athleticism. Other than your typical, 1 gram of protein per bodyweight bodybuilding rule of thumb, I will list some valid studies below.

- Research conducted by scientists at McMaster University. According to their work, protein intake of 1.3 to 1.8 grams per kilogram of body weight (0.6 to 0.8 grams per pound of body weight) is adequate for stimulating maximal protein synthesis. We can derive that more protein may be needed in the case of frequent and/ or high-intensity training and or in the case of dieting in an attempt to lose fat (restricting calories)[26].

- Auckland University of Technology: "Protein needs for energy-restricted resistance-trained athletes are likely 2.3-3.1g/ kg of FFM [1 - 1.4 grams per pound of fat free mass] scaled upwards with severity of caloric restriction and leanness." Your fat free mas can be calculated by taking your body weight and multiplying it by your body fat percentage {(Weight*BF%=Fat Weight)-Weight=Fat Free Mass)} calculated by taking your body fat percentage and subtracting it from your body weight. Subtract your fat weight from your body weight and you have your lean body mass[19].

The first Hercules (Steeve Reeves) ate roughly 164 grams of protein per day and weighed 220lbs. Personally I have found that I develop strength and size with a diet that is 3530% protein. That is counting the protein in my carbohydrate, and fat sources as well. The method of multiplying my protein needs by 1-1.4 grams per fat free mass works well with me as well as clients. I even "shred-up" the best on that low of protein because my body is getting all the correct nutrients it needs to function at optimal rates.

Now we can work on what whole foods to eat so you can grow or loose while flourishing. First, we will need to understand some principles of your macronutrient sources:

Not all Proteins Are Created Equal

Many IFYM dieters and vegetarians or vegans believe that all proteins are created equal. This is incorrect. Remember, amino acids are the building blocks of protein? Your body needs 22 different types of amino acids to function properly. Adults can synthesize 13 of those within the body (known as non-essential amino acids), but the other 9 must be obtained from food (known as essential amino acids)[29]. When you look on the back of a bag of broccoli, there is about 3g of protein for 1-cup serving. It's a lot of protein per serving but it is not a complete source of protein per serving because broccoli does not contain enough essential amino acids per serving. Take a look at a comparison of broccoli compared to steak below.

Essential Amino acids (g)	Daily requirement 70 kg adult (g)	Essential amino acids (g) in 275 calories of steak (4 oz or 113.33 g)	Essential amino acids (g) in raw 277 calories of chopped, broccoli (9.25 cups)
histidine	0.70	0.975 (+0.275)	0.48 (-0.22)
isoleucine	1.400	1.391 (-0.009)	0.643 (-0.757)
leucine	2.730	2.431 (-0.299)	1.05 (-1.68)
lysine	2.100	2.583 (+0.483)	1.099 (-1.001)
methionine	0.70	0.796 (+0.096)	0.309 (-0.391)
cysteine	0.28	0.394 (+ 0.114)	0.228 (-0.052)
threonine	1.050	1.221 (+0.171)	0.716 (-0.334)
tryptophan	0.280	0.201 (-0.079)	0.269 (-0.011)
valine	1.82	1.516 (-0.304)	1.018 (-0.802)

*https://eathropology.com/2013/04/08/broccoli-has-more-protein-than-steak-and-other-crap/

According to the USDA's Agricultural Research Service's Nutrient Data Laboratory database, 100 calories of broiled beef, top sirloin steak has *exactly* 11.08 grams of protein and 100 calories of chopped, raw broccoli has *exactly* 8.29. Not only does steak have more protein than broccoli but it has a lot more essential amino acids needed for protein synthesis. "It would be difficult to find a protein that does not have at least one residue of each of the common 20 amino acids. Half of these amino acids are essential, and *if the diet is lacking or low in even one of these essential amino acids, then protein synthesis is not possible*" [Emphasis mine; reference: Campbell & Farrell's Biochemistry, 6th edition]. Guess what guys? Protein synthesis is needed for growth, muscle repair/building, and general body function.

-Complete Sources of Protein:

Pure	Meat	Dairy	Complete Grain	Grain & Lentils (Vegetarian)	Grain & Dairy (Vegetarian)
Protein Powder (Isolate)	Fish (crab, shrimp & lobster included)	Greek-Yogurt (Plain is a lot healthier)	Quinoa	Brown Rice and Red Beans	Steel Cut Oates & Milk
Egg Whites	Poultry: Chicken & Turkey	Milk (Any Fat Grade)	Ezekiel Bread	Barley & Lentils	Bread & Cheese
	Eggs	Cheese (The harder the cheese the better)	Soybean	Hummus (Chickpeas) & Whole Grain Pita	Whole Grain Cereal & Milk
	Lean Beef	Cottage Cheese	Ground Flaxseed	Peanut Butter & Whole Grain Crackers	
				Whole Grain Pasta & Milk or Cheese	
				Corn & Black Beans	

Know that we know how to combine different food sources to create a complete protein we can kind of figure this whole eating thing out. Well hold up. For those of you who are trying to maximize your full potential with protein you must understand this. Some proteins sources have a higher absorbable rate than others.

Food Source	Percentage of Protein Utilization
Eggs	94
Milk (Whey & Casein Protein Powders)	82
Fish	80
Cheese	70
Brown Rice	70
Meat & Poultry	68
Soybean Flour	61

18

What can we take from this table? There is a big difference of how much protein a food source contains and how much you can use to actually build muscle. We can also see that supplemented protein drinks are not the best source of protein. Boom, to all of you supplement companies out there shoving protein powders and pills down peoples. Sorry to all of those people like me who have been tricked for some time. I will even make a protein rating chart listed by amino acid absorption from best to worst with eggs being of quality 100:

Food Source	Protein Rating
Eggs	100
Fish	70
Milk	69
Lean Beef	69

Soybeans	47
Dry Beans	34
Whole-Grain Wheat	44

A healthy diet will have a protein sources from all groups, but you may pick and choose depending on your liking. Personally, my physique looks best when I eliminate all protein powders for pure egg whites. That means no processed carbohydrates, whey protein after the gym, and no casein shake at night.

Carbohydrates

We have already gone into details about carbohydrates. Have you ever dropped your carbs to "shred up" but your weight training sucks, energy levels are low, your mood sucks, you can't think, and you lose a lot of your size? Here's why. Carbs, the body's main source of energy, are stored in the muscles as glycogen, which helps fuel the most intense weight training sessions. Carbs also have a "protein-sparing" effect that keeps our bodies from burning up protein for energy. Protein can be converted to carbs in the liver but carbs cannot be converted to protein. Deprivation of carbs can have severe side effects on mood, thought process, and personality. Remember not all carbs are created equal. Some carbs are slower digesting while others digest faster.

Fats

Fats are a truly amazing macronutrient, especially for men. They can be found in both plant source and animal source foods. Fats are a major source of stored energy. When you think of a grizzly bear preparing for hibernation, you think of a bear eating and getting fat for the winter right? The bears eat so much in summer in attempt to store body fat for the cold winters. Our bodies work the same way. Our fat storage works in the same manner because we naturally store fats for body heat. Fat also provides necessary cushion for organs in our bodies.

Remember, fats contain the most calorie per gram. A pound of body fat roughly contains 3,500 calories (same as a pound of muscle). The general conception is, if I eat fats, I will get fat. This is not the case as you should have a diet that is 20-30% in fat. If you choose to go any lower in fat intake your fat loss may come to a halt, recovery times will stint, and hormonal levels and testosterone levels will drop. I once did a 1990's lowfat (15% or under) bodybuilding diet with medium protein, and high carb diet; I gained 20 lb's within 3 months and I had a lot of energy, but when it came to the bedroom, I had no drive at all. Point is, your ability to produce testosterone is highly dependent on your dietary fat intake.

Your fat intake should be highly comprised of unsaturated and monosaturated. These types of fats include flaxseed, sunflower, olive oil, canola oil, fish oil, and nuts. If you happen to saturated fats, it okay as you need about 10% of your fat to be saturated for cholesterol purposes. A certain amount of cholesterol (daily range of 250-500) is healthy and is needed for healthy testosterone. You may find it in foods such as eggs, steak, chicken, milk, coconut oil, butter, and cheese. Steer completely away from trans-fat as it is a processed man-made fat and they damage your cellular system. Examples of trans fat include corn oil, chips, bottled salad dressings, deep-fat fried foods, doughnuts, margarine and more. So stay away from "junk"!

Micronutrients

"Above all don't worry. Worry brings fear and fear is crippling. The only thing that can cause you to worry is trying this journey all by yourself. Know that all you have to do is hold your goal before you. Everything else will take care of itself." -Jim Rohn

Micronutrients are substances that the body needs in small amounts that we get while eating our food. Vitamins, minerals, and water account for the micronutrients in the body. There is no energy or fat loss contribution from vitamins, but help promote reactions in your body. Let me explain the two different sources of vitamins. I have a weird and awkward question for you, have you ever urinated and your pee may be greenish after taking a multi-vitamin? If so, it's because your body is flushing out watersoluble vitamins. Water soluble vitamins are not stored in your body and are needed from food sources. Any excess water soluble vitamins are flushed out while urinating. On the other hand, fat-soluble vitamins are unneeded on a daily basis and are stored in our bodies' fat tissue.

-Water-Soluble Vitamins

B6(pyridoxine), B1 (thiamine), B2 (riboflavin), Niacin, Pantothenic acid, Biotin, Choline

Folacin (folic acid), B12 (cyanocobalamin), & Vitamin C (ascorbic acid)

Vitamin B1- Helps promote a healthy nervous system and helps your body utilize carbohydrates at their maximum benefit. This vitamin can be found in lentils, black beans, sunflower seeds, and...

Vitamin B2- Assist in healthy skin and helps your body breakdown macronutrients. This vitamin can be found in milk

Niacin- Assist in energy production and maintaining a healthy digestive and nervous system. This vitamin can be found in chicken, turkey, halibut, and tuna.

Pantothenic acid- Aids in assist in protein synthesis and sustaining life. This vitamin can be found in fish, milk, eggs, avocados, legumes and yams.

Biotin- Assist in maintaining a healthy red blood supply by maximizing the use of other nutrients. This vitamin can be found in small doses in legumes, tomatoes, romaine lettuce, and almonds.

Choline- Assists in liver function, brain development, nerve function, and metabolism. Choline can be found in eggs, liver, beef, salmon, cauliflower, and brussel sprouts.

Folic Acid- Assist in the reproduction of new cells and the prevention of anemia. This vitamin can be found in lentils, beans, asparagus, and spinach.

Vitamin B12- Is important in DNA synthesis. This vitamin can be found in meat, fish, and dairy. It is very common to see a vegan diet lacking this necessary vitamin because it is only found in animal products.

Vitamin C- Contains antioxidants that assist in a safe immune system and assist in marinating proper connective tissue in both your cartilage and tendons. Vitamin C can be found in most fruits and there is an abundant source in broccoli and brussel sprouts.

-Fat-Soluble Vitamins:

Vitamin A, Vitamin D, Vitamin E, & Vitamin K

I won't describe the Fat-Soluble vitamins since they are unneeded on a daily basis and stored in the body for long periods of time.

Minerals play a big role in one's diet. If you are eating a variety of meats and vegetables, you should be consuming an adequate amount of minerals. First hand, I can tell you that when you do consume protein sources from different meats and you are eating a variety of vegetables, your body will transform. Last, but not least, is water.

Water is one of the most important components of the body. Our bodies are made up of 50-75% water. Remember our talk about glycogen in your muscles getting bigger? Part of the reason behind this is water; our muscles are made up of 72% water. Do you ever see those meatheads at the gym carrying around their big gallon water bottles? There is a reason why they do that. Water and hydration assist in increased blood volume and fluid to fill your veins and arteries with nutrients. The greater the nutrients, the greater the muscle and "pump" effect. One to two gallons of water a day is adequate depending on training and carbohydrate intake. For food digestion purposes, it is best to drink your water 30 minutes after eating and 30 minutes before eating. I just want to clarify this now; you do not need amino acids in your gallon water jug. If you are eating a rich protein diet you will have more than enough protein to stay in an anabolic (growth) muscle state. Where their amino acid powders in the 50's and 60's?

Dairy Products

Yogurt does aid the digestive process by stimulating the colon, but only a teaspoon a week is needed to aid with your intensive health[7]. For bodybuilders and physique builders, a diet high in yogurt and dairy can ruin some of the best training programs in the world. Yogurt tends to cause a layer of fat to form beneath the skin and results in a lack of definition at low body fat levels. I realized this while experimenting with my diet before my second competition. I eliminated milk, Greek yogurt, and protein powders, all of which had dairy, and my skin was a lot tighter. I do not recommend eliminating dairy from your diet unless you are allergic, are trying to go to Vegas during the summer to show off your new physique, or if you are competing. In this case, you would want to eliminate it from your diet one or two months before. Otherwise, you can still achieve an astonishing looking and healthy body while consuming dairy.

Muscle Building Supplements

He who takes medicine and neglects to diet wastes the skill of his doctors - Chinese Proverb

What comes to mind when someone in the gym asks you about supplements? Protein powders, pre-workout, creatine, amino acids (aminos), fat burning accelerators, pills, powders, liquids, and maybe even steroids. News flash- none of the supplements is needed for weight loss, nor muscle growth. Protein powders may be necessary to fulfill your daily intake of protein if you did not have time to prepare your food or if you have none in your vicinity. Otherwise don't waste your time because these muscle building supplements are more harmful for you than they are good and they are not regulated by the Federal Food and Drug commission. Trust me, I know, I started a supplement company trying to "make it" following my passion. I dropped the business after I figured out that supplements are more harmful for the human body than they are good. I wanted to help people, not hurt them. People associate supplements with hot fitness models and ripped muscle models. I have buddies that got sponsors, but I wanted no part. My model of growth has always been Natty or natural. The roided-outlook has never appealed to me. Plus, I've never been the type to be a cheater.

Whey and Casein protein are derivatives of cow's milk. Whey is more of a fast digesting protein that is more likely to spike your insulin after a work out because its speed of digestion. There are so many whey proteins in the market, which makes it hard to make a choice if you HAVE TO find one that is the purest and most digestible. Quality does matter when it comes to protein powder. Casein protein is basically processed cottage cheese. It digests very slowly because of the size and construction of the protein. Many supplement companies say take it before bed so you stay anabolic all night. I have tried this for many years, and casein powder bloats you and can cause some serious digestive issues. If you want a quality protein before bed, try egg whites. Egg whites provide you with all the necessary protein you need without all the added sucralose, maltodextrin, cellulose gum, and artificial flavors. If you're a 'whatever it takes' type of person, eat your egg whites, not the powder.

When you think of creatine, you think of crystalized powder and water filled muscles. Let's take a look at what creatine is and how it was first discovered. Creatine is a natural substance, meaning your body already produces it, stored in your muscle cells used for a 10-15 second energy burst. By supplementing with creatine, you may provide yourself with a more powerful workout. Creatine pulls water from your body into your muscle cells to increase volumization while working out; hence, you get a better and bigger pump and a bigger look. Creatine powder emerged in the early 1990's because bodybuilders like Leroy

Colbert (21" arms) would go and eat steak and potatoes after their workout. The bodybuilders that followed this routine found out that they felt more powerful in their following workouts. When they ate chicken, instead of steak, their workouts were not as powerful and volumizing.

Looking further into this, scientist found that red meat contained a source of energy called creatine. Nowadays, creatine is derived from red meat and sold in powdered forms. Guys and gals, let me let you in on a little secret. You can get all the added natural creatine you need to provide yourself with a more powerful workout by eating lean steak before or after your workout or both. This prevents the chance of overdosing on creatine and damaging your kidneys and liver.

Branch-Chain Amino Acids (BCAA) are made up of the three essential amino acids leucine, isoleucine, and valine. These amino acids cannot be synthesized by the body, meaning your body cannot produce them. I will tell you once again, don't waste your money. The best sources of BCAAs are meat, chicken, fish, dairy products and eggs, reports NYU Langone Medical Center. If you want your BCAAs during or after your workout, eat chicken breast or eggs before your workout and steak after. Your body will take some time to digest your source of protein before your workout (BCAAs during your workout) and you will get your added creatine/BCAA benefits after your workout from eating steak. Try it out.

Glutamine is an amino acid that is marketed and sold as one of the most important muscle building amino acids. You usually start by taking 5grams after your workout. I've tried this and it didn't work. Again, sources of amino acids are important to build a protein for muscle growth. Glutamine makes up approximately 50-60% of the free amino acids in muscle, but it is also a non-essential amino acid[26]. I took glutamine for years until I came across a study in my American College of Exercise Trainers Manual. The study revealed that there were no added benefits to athletes that took glutamine after their exercise routine. Guess what? Supplementary glutamine is unnecessary because our body already produces it.

Carnitine is a newly marketed amino acid that is claimed to be an added benefit for energy, muscle building, and fat burning. L-carnitine supplements are used to increase carnitine levels in people whose natural level of carnitine is too low because they have a genetic disorder, are taking certain drugs (valproic acid for seizures), or because they are undergoing a medical procedure (hemodialysis for kidney disease) that uses up the body's L-carnitine. Unless you have a genetic disease that causes you seizures to where you do not synthesize the non-essential amino acid carnitine, you don't need to supplement with carnitine and its other forms.

Pre-workout was already explained in the myths section of this game plan.

A major ingredient in today's pre-workout is beta-alanine. Beta-alanine is another nonessential amino acid. Beta-alanine is used for improving athletic performance and exercise capacity, building lean muscle mass and improving physical functioning in the elderly. Webmd.com says that, beta-alanine is **Possibly Safe** when taken for a short time and side effects have not been reported with moderate doses [3]. High doses of betaalanine can cause flushing and tingling. Sound and feel familiar? That itching and tingling feeling is called "paresthesia" which correlates with disorders of the brain, spinal cord, and peripheral nerves[21]. Nowadays, pre-workout is loaded with betaalanine. Heck, most will even put "loaded" on the label.

Now for the big one, Caffeine. Caffeine is a stimulant to your brain and central nervous system. Caffeine delays fatigue and increases mental and physical activity. This forces your body to use emergency reserves that should be replenished by rest. If you think a cup of coffee or a pre-workout is good before your workout, think again. Caffeine triggers a flow of stimulating chemicals from the adrenal glands in your brain into your bloodstream, causing your blood sugar levels to spike (bad). The rise of blood sugar levels causes your blood vessels to contract and raise blood pressure up to 10 percent[7].

When caffeine is used on a regular basis, it causes a mild physical dependence. If you stop taking your caffeine you may develop several withdraw symptoms which include: headache, fatigue, anxiety, irritability, depressed mood, and difficulty concentrating. Sounds familiar? Have you ever stopped taking your pre-workout for a period of time? Most likely, you developed the same symptoms. Pre-workout is loaded with caffeine so you can adapt a physical dependence. Then you will never workout without your preworkout. Too much caffeine in one sitting will literally make you heart explode. Seriously, I know many of supplement/energy drink in lawsuits over caffeine and other stimulants blowing up people's hearts. I won't throw out any names; you can do your own research.

*Remember, before you say, "whatever it takes", "I don't care, I just want to get big now", "I don't care, I just want to slim down or shred up now", a good looking body is a healthy body.

Recommended Supplements for Health & Muscle Growth

"Sell yourself short on nutrition and you're selling yourself short on maximizing your physique development." -
Ernie Taylor

Let's face it; athletes' bodies do take a beating. Whether you a triathlon, professional football player, strongman, or bodybuilder, your body will take a toll. Many runners and athletes die early because they sweat out and expend the necessary nutrients in their bodies and never refuel them. Below are some supplements that I recommend to supplement with a nutrient rich diet.

- Zinc: U.S. soil is low in this mineral which aids with fingernails, hair, skin, digestive, metabolism, and prostate gland health.

- Calcium/Magnesium: Calcium aids with the prevention of cramps, blood clots, and is needed for the breakdown of protein molecules. Magnesium aids with the conversion of blood sugar into energy; hence, it activates enzymes needed for muscular energy. When these two minerals work together, they help maintain strong bones and teeth.

- Vitamin C: Will assist in building collagen, fighting off infections and will help boost immune system. Vitamin C is necessary for teeth, bones and the formation of red blood cells.

- Vitamin D3: Aids with the regulation of your metabolism and absorption of cramps.

- Multivitamin: Will work as an aid to receive all of your recommend vitamins and minerals that you do not receive from your food.

- Vitamin B12: Regulates a healthy nervous system and metabolism. Is also essential to normal maturation of red blood cells which prevents anemia.

- Digestive Enzymes: If you have digestive issues, this will aid in the digestion of nutrients.

Alcohol

Many of us use alcohol as a way to escape conflicts, to cope, to be cool with your friends, or to alter or state of conciseness. Alcohol is high in calories, especially hard liquor, and it will induce muscle dehydration. If you must drink alcohol in moderation, beer or wine should be your choice. Beer is low in sugar aid wine contains over 300 enzymes that promote digestion of fats and proteins. Your body will utilize a small amount of alcohol effectively; therefore, if you do decide to consume alcohol with your daily nutrition you should drink no more than eight ounces of wine or beer daily. Four ounces at lunch and four ounces at dinner is doable with eight ounces of water in each serving.

If you are using alcohol as a coping method, it will damage your health and you will lose your muscle mass. I fell into this trap of using alcohol and even chewing Tabaco while trying to maintain an image. I decided to replace this coping method with exercise and bodybuilding. My progress shot up considerably and I felt a night and day difference in health and energy.

Intermittent Fasting

The new and cool principle of intermittent fasting is hot. Truth is, it has always been there. You do it every night. Intermittent fasting isn't a fad diet; instead, it is a period of time where you eat your calories during a specific window of the day, and choosing not to eat food during the rest. With intermittent fasting, you may choose the periods you eat and the ones you don't eat. You can choose 8a.m.-4p.m. (8-hour window), 12p.m.-6p.m. (6-hour window), and a 10a.m.-2p.m. Since studies show you can burn the same amount of calories in eating a couple meals a day rather than spreading all of your calories out, the eating method of intermittent fasting is a new hit. You basically fit all of your macronutrients in during which ever period of time you choose. Some even skip meals for 24 hours and then you eat twice as much the next day.

Although you can lose just of much fat eating this method rather than spreading your meals out for hours, this can be done but it just sounds insane because you will lose muscle, feel like trash for hours upon hours, and you will be tired with a loss of focus for a long period of time. This should only be the case if you are competing in a bodybuilding show, otherwise it's not recommended. If you want to try it, you already are. Your body goes through an intermittent fasting and burns fat for energy while you sleep. So if someone asks, "Hey bud, you're looking shredded. Are you doing intermittent fasting?" Say, "Yeah, man I invented it and I've been doing it for years now. Where have you been?"

Chapter Twelve: Eating for a Successful Life

"Don't live to eat, eat to live" -Your Author

I will list a couple of meal plans below for males and females. A meal plan "coach" or "guru" will usually cost you around $300 a month. But, there is a reason why you are reading this book. It's because you're a do-it-yourselfer. After you read this section, you will be quite aware of what to eat to gain or lose fat. I will only ask one favor in return and I will list it at the end of this section.

These programs will depend solely on your schedule and your metabolism. If you often feel hungry, you may want to eat at least 5 meals a day. No, the method of spreading your calories throughout the day does not boost your metabolism, but it does have some added benefits. I also recommend more meals per day because you can assemble your protein sources better and you can assemble your carbohydrates without spiking your insulin levels, so you are less likely to add body fat. This is not a one size fits all plan, because the amount of calories you eat depends on your metabolism, activity level, muscle mass, and goals. In order to build a strong and healthy looking body, it is not about how much you eat, but it is about what you eat. Therefore, I will only list nutrient dense foods in these sample diet plans. Remember, sculpting your body or building your body should be sustainable, healthy, and long lasting.

Meal Plans

Lean Muscle Building Plan- (160lb Male) (45% Carbs, 35% Protein, 20% Fats)

Breakfast:

1 Large Brown Egg

3/4 Cup Egg Whites

1 Steel Cut Microwavable Oates (Add Cinnamon for Flavor)

Cup Fat Free Milk (Water May be Used if Non-Dairy)

½ Cup Blueberries

Fish Oil Pills

1 Multi Vitamin, 1000mg of Vitamin C, 5000 IU Vitamin D3, 1 Cal/Mag Tablet, 1000mg HMB

Post-Workout Meal:

1 Scoop of Isolate Protein (Iso Sensation 93 or Iso-100)

1 Cup Jasmin Rice

5 grams of creatine

1000 grams HMB

Meal 3:

1 Cup Non-Fat Greek Yogurt

1 Cup Raspberries or Blackberries or Mix

1 Tbsp Natural Honey

10 Almonds or Hazelnuts

         Or (Non-Dairy)

5 oz Tilapia

5 oz Yam (With Cinnamon)

5 oz Asparagus (Drizzled with Lemon Juice)

10 Almonds or Hazelnuts

Meal 4:

3oz. Chicken Breast

1 Cup Chopped Broccoli or Green Beans or Brussel sprouts

1 Cup Long-Grain Brown Rice

½ Cup of Cooked Lentils or Chickpeas

Meal 5:

6 oz. Sockeye Salmon

6oz Yam (Add Cinnamon for Flavor)

5oz Asparagus (Use Liquid Amino Acid Soy Sauce Alternative for Flavor or Lemon Juice)

Before Bed (Keep your body burning fat for energy while you sleep):

Cup Egg Whites or ¾ Cup of Fat Free Cottage Cheese

Tbsp Natural Almond Butter or Peanut Butter or 4oz Avocado

2 Fish Oil Pills

1000mg HMB

Average Daily total: 2,456 calories, 208 grams protein, 266 grams carbohydrates, 59 grams of fat

Lean Muscle Growth Plan with Fat Loss- (Female) (Roughly 50% Carbs, 30% Protein, 20% Fats)

Breakfast

1 Slice of Ezekiel Bread (Spread Nutt Butter or Avocado)

1 Large Brown Egg

¾ Cup Egg Whites

1 Cup Spinach

1 Tbsp of Natural Peanut Butter or Almond Butter or 2 oz of Avocado

1 Grapefruit

1 Fish Oil Pill

1 Multi Vitamin, 1000mg of Vitamin C, 5000 IU Vitamin D3, 1 Cal/Mag Tablet, 1000 mg HMB

Post-Workout Meal

¾ Scoop of Iso protein

1 Cup Jasmin Rice

        Or

3/4 Scoop of Iso protein

Plain Rice Cakes (Smoother Baby Food on Rice Cakes)

TBSP Baby Food (No Fat & No Fiber)

Meal 3

3oz 99% Lean Ground Turkey or Chicken Breast

½ Cup of Brown Rice

1/3 Cup Black Beans (Eat Non-Tinned as they Have a Lower-GI)

½ Lime

1 Cup Spinach

Meal 4

4oz Tilapia or Cod or Ahi Tuna

6oz Yams with Cinnamon

4oz Broccoli or Green Beans or Brussel Sprouts Drizzled with Lemon Juice (Lemon is a Natural Antioxidant)

Meal 5

4oz 96% Lean Beef or Top Sirloin or Eye of Round Steak

¾ Cup Quinoa

5oz Steamed Asparagus or Broccoli Drizzled with Lemon Juice

Late Night Snack

½ Cup Fat-Free Cottage Cheese or ¾ cup egg whites

1 Tbsp Natural Peanut Butter or Almond Butter or 2oz Avocado

Fish Oil Pill

1000mg HMB

Average Daily total: 1,836 calories, 154 grams protein, 231 grams carbohydrates, 36 grams of fat

Fat Loss & Muscle Growth- (210 lb. Male) (Roughly 40% Carbs, 40% Protein, & 20% Fat)

Breakfast

1 Slices of Ezekiel Bread (Breakfast Sandwich)

2 oz Avocado

1 Large Brown Egg

3/4 Cup Egg Whites

1 Cup Spinach

3 Fish Oil Pills

Multi Vitamin, 1000mg of Vitamin C, 5000 IU Vitamin D3, 1 Cal/Mag Tablet, 1000mg HMB

Post Workout

1.25 Scoop Iso Protein (Iso-Sensation 93 or Iso-100)

35 oz of Sports Drink

Meal 3

6 oz Sockeye Salmon

5oz Asparagus (Drizzled with Lemon Juice)

Meal 4

4 oz Boneless Chicken Breast

1 Cup Quinoa

oz Asparagus (Drizzled with Lemon Juice)

Meal 5

oz Tilapia or Cod or Mui Tuna

6 oz Yam (Add Cinnamon for Flavor)

6 oz Broccoli (Use Liquid Amino Acid Soy Sauce Alternative for Flavor)

Before Bed

Cup Egg Whites

Tbsp Natural Peanut Butter or Almond Butter or 4 oz Avocado

Fish Oil Pills

1000mg HMB

Average Daily total: 1,836 calories, 182 grams protein, 184 grams carbohydrates, 54 grams of fat *Depending on your time of training, morning or night, you may switch up your post workout meal. For example, switch post workout meal for meal 5 for men and meal 4 for woman. All meats should be trimmed and weighed before cooking. All carb sources are weighed after cooking except for steel-cut oats and vegetables.

Now, that I provided you with a healthy and truthful non fad way of losing/gaining weight, I ask a favor in return. I ask that you go and write a great review from wherever you purchased this book. My goal is to benefit and share this information with as many people as possible. I want to help as many people that want to be helped. I want to help those who are looking for the truth. I want to help those who are looking for answers. Yes, they have to buy it, but it's a lot cheaper than hiring a trainer or paying for a meal prep plan. Plus, there is value in things you buy and people are more likely to stick to it.

Chapter Thirteen: What You Will Need on Your New Journey

Along with a successful attitude and new bound knowledge, you will need a couple additives to make things a lot easier day-to-day and year-to-year.

1. Food scale- A simple electronic food scale allows you to weigh all of your food. This item can be purchased at just about any general merchandise retailer.
2. Sport watch- A sport watch comes in handy during rest periods in between sets. It sure does beat counting in your head or starring at the clock. A simple sport watch can be purchased at just about any general merchandise retailer.
3. Meal bag- Do you bring your lunch pail to work? Well, this is the same concept. You will need a bag to carry around all of your meals for the day. If not, you will most likely skip a meal or run to the fast food joint. There are several meal prep bag companies out there nowadays. Just type it into your search engine and there you go.
4. Grocery List- Just like you come prepared to the gym with a workout in mind, you must go to the grocery store with the same mentality. It all starts with a solid plan and a grocery list is a solid plan for your nutrient needs. I have attached a sample grocery list in the back of this book for you.
5. Water Jug- If you decide to carry a gallon around and people make fun of you, oh well. They will be doing the same thing in a couple of years when they realize the true benefit of the miracle drink, water. Stay healthy, stay hydrated!
6. Pencil- You will need to take a pencil with you to the gym to record your weight and progress in the back of this book. Tracking your progress is very important. Plus, it feels good to say, "I was here and I got here that quick".

Endnote: There is So Much More to Life

"There's more to life than training, but training is what puts more in your life." - Brooks Kubik

To all of you youngsters out there reading this or even those in their twenties, there is so much more to life other than training. You may want to start a family, travel the world, or even start a business to help others. Don't let yourself fall into the trap of training and going home and resting to do it all over again. Look forward to other things in life and don't make it your only. Working out and eating healthy requires an enormous amount of discipline and time in life, but it will better the quality your life.

Bibliography:

1. Adkins, W. D. "Aerobic & Anaerobic Heart Rate Zones." *LIVESTRONG.COM.* LIVESTRONG.COM, 08 June 2015. Web. 20 Aug. 2016.
2. "American Heart Association Recommendations for Physical Activity in Adults." *American Heart Association Recommendations for Physical Activity in Adults.* N.p., 1 Feb. 2014. Web. 20 Aug. 2016.
3. Athletes: A Case for Higher Intakes," International Journal of Sport Nutrition and Exercise Metabolism 24, no. 2 (2014): 127-38. doi: 10.1123/ ijsnem. 2013-0054.
4. "BETA-ALANINE: Uses, Side Effects, Interactions and Warnings - WebMD." *WebMD.* WebMD, n.d. Web. 20 Aug. 2016.
5. "Calcium Levels in Milk vs. Almond, Rice and Soy Milk / Nutrition / Healthy Eating." *Calcium Levels in Milk vs. Almond, Rice and Soy Milk / Nutrition / Healthy Eating.* Fitday Editor, n.d. Web. 20 Aug. 2016.
6. Chriss, James J. "The Functions Of The Social Bond." *Sociological Quarterly The Sociological Quarterly* 48.4 (2007): 689-712. Web.
7. Columbu, Franco, and Lydia Fragomeni. *The Bodybuilder's Nutrition Book.* Chicago: Contemporary, 1985. Print.
8. Dallas, Marry E. "The Best High-Fiber Foods for Lower Cholesterol." *EverydayHealth.com.* Nivya Jones, n.d. Web. 20 Aug. 2016.
9. Eric R. Helms, Caryn Zinn, David S. Rowlands, and Scott R. Brown, "A Systematic Review of
10. Dietary Protein during Caloric Restriction in Resistance Trained Lean
11. "Fitness." *Fitness.* Yash Goel, n.d. Web. 20 Aug. 2016.
12. Girad, Hugo. "6 Pack Lapadat." *6 Pack Lapadat.* N.p., n.d. Web. 20 Aug. 2016.
13. Hansen, John. *Natural Bodybuilding.* 1st ed. Vol. 1. Australia: Human Kenetics, 2005. Print.
14. Hite, Adele. "Eathropology." *Eathropology.* N.p., 08 Apr. 2013. Web. 20 Aug. 2016.
15. "Hyponatremia." - *Mayo Clinic.* Ed. Mayo Clinic Staff. Mayo Clinic, 28 May 2014. Web. 20 Aug. 2016.
16. Jesse. "The Best Exercises For Legs – 5 KILLER Exercises to Build up Your Legs!" *Truth Of Building Muscle.* N.p., Nov.-Dec. 2014. Web. 20 Aug. 2016.
17. Keller, Gary, and Jay Papasan. *The One Thing: The Surprisingly Simple Truth behind Extraordinary Results.* Austin, TX: Bard, 2012. Print.
18. Lapadat, Ryan. "Exercise Images." *6 Pack Lapadat Pro Strongman.* N.p., n.d. Web. 20 Aug. 2016.
19. Marker, Craig. "Use Eccentric Movements to Build Strength and Improve Flexibility." *Breaking Muscle.* N.p., n.d. Web. 20 Aug. 2016.
20. Marrow, Nate. "List of Complete vs. Incomplete Protein Sources - BuiltLean." *BuiltLean.* N.p., 03 Oct. 2012. Web. 20 Aug. 2016

21. "MUSCLES MOTIVATION – Photos." *MUSCLES MOTIVATION*. N.p., n.d. Web. 20 Aug. 2016.

22. "NINDS Paresthesia Information Page." *Paresthesia Information Page: National Institute of Neurological Disorders and Stroke (NINDS)*. Office of Communications and Public Liaison, 11 Sept. 2015. Web. 20 Aug. 2016.

23. Nuckols, Greg. "Gender Differences in Training and Metabolism • Strengtheory." *Strengtheory*. N.p., 11 Jan. 2015. Web. 21 Aug. 2016.

24. Park, Madison. "Twinkie Diet Helps Nutrition Professor Lose 27 Pounds." *CNN*. Cable News Network, 08 Nov. 2010. Web. 20 Aug. 2016.

25. Roth E, et al. (1990). Glutamine: anabolic effector? Journal Parent Ent Nutrition. 14: 1305-65.

26. Schwarzenegger, Arnold, and Bill Dobbins. *Encyclopedia of Modern Bodybuilding*. London: Pelham, 1985. Print.

27. Stuart M. Phillips and Luc J. C. Van Loon, "Dietary Protein for Athletes: From Requirements to Optimum Adaptation," Journal of Sports Sciences 29, no. S1 (2011): S29-S38. doi: 10.1080/ 02640414.2011.619204.

28. The complete list of the glycemic index and glycemic load for more than 1,000 foods can be found in the article "International tables of glycemic index and glycemic load values:

29. 2008" by Fiona S. Atkinson, Kaye Foster-Powell, and Jennie C. Brand-Miller in the December 2008 issue of Diabetes Care, Vol. 31, number 12, pages 2281-2283.

30. "The Difference Between Meat, Soy, Whey, Dairy, and Vegan Types of Protein." *Comparison of Meat, Soy, Whey, Dairy, and Vegan Types of Protein*. N.p., n.d. Web. 07 Sept. 2016.

31. "You Searched for Muscle+group - Fitneass." *Fitneass*. N.p., n.d. Web. 20 Aug. 2016.

32. Zuhl, Michah, and Len Kravitz. "HIIT vs. Continuous Cardiovascular Exercise." *HIIT vs. Continuous Cardiovascular Exercise*. N.p., n.d. Web. 20 Aug. 2016.

Part VI: Body Engineering Tools

Nutrient Dense Grocery List

Protein Sources:

1. Eye of Round Steak Trimmed or 96% Lean Ground Beef
2. Boneless Chicken Breast
3. 99% Lean Ground Turkey
4. Soybeans (Pasta) = 21g
5. Lentils (Incomplete Protein) = 18g
6. Black Beans = 15g
7. Chickpeas AKA Gonzo Bean (Incomplete Add Rice, Bread, or Quinoa)= 12 g
8. Baked Beans (Incomplete) = 12g
9. Quinoa = 9g
10. Peanut or Almond Butter = 8g
11. Ezekiel Bread = 4g
12. Hummus and Pita (Incomplete Add Rice or Wheat) = 7g
13. Eggs (Brown Vegan Fed) or Egg Whites
14. Nonfat plain Greek Yogurt
15. Fish (Ahi Tuna, Tilapia, Cod, & Wild Salmon)

Calcium Source (1,000g Needed):

1. Nonfat Milk
2. Nonfat Greek Yogurt Plain (or dairy products)
3. Cal/Mag Tablet

Vegetables:

1. Broccoli
2. Kale
3. Spinach
4. Collard Greens
5. Asparagus
6. Brussel Sprouts
7. Green Beans
8. Garlic
9. Mushroom
10. Tomato
11. Cabbage
12. Lemon/Lime

Fruits:

1. Apple (Organic Less Pesticides)
2. Banana
3. Blueberries
4. Raspberries (Low Sugar Highest in Fiber)
5. Blackberries (Low Sugar)
6. Grapefruit/Orange

Fats & Oils:

1. Avocado
2. Raw Almonds
3. Flaxseed (Ground or Oil)
4. Chia seeds ({Don't Recommend will bloat you if you eat too much} it's just a marketing scheme)
5. Olive oil cooking spray
6. Canola oil cooking spray
7. Raw Peanuts or Natural Peanut Butter
8. Walnuts
9. Fish Oil (Salmon or Supplement)
10. Egg Yolk

Vitamin B-12:

1. Brewers and Nutritional Yeast
2. Supplement

Strachey Low-GI Carbohydrate Sources:

1. Steel Cut Oats
2. Yam
3. Brown Rice
4. Barilla Plus Noodle or Soybean Noodles
5. Quinoa
6. Barley
7. Cuscus

Glycemic Index Chart

FOOD	Glycemic index (glucose = 100)	Serving size (grams)	Glycemic load per serving
BAKERY PRODUCTS AND BREADS			
Banana cake, made with sugar	47	60	14
Banana cake, made without sugar	55	60	12
Sponge cake, plain	46	63	17
Vanilla cake made from packet mix with vanilla frosting (Betty Crocker)	42	111	24
Apple muffin, made with rolled oats and sugar	44	60	13
Apple muffin, made with rolled oats and without sugar	48	60	9
Waffles, Aunt Jemima®	76	35	10
Bagel, white, frozen	72	70	25
Baguette, white, plain	95	30	14
Coarse barley bread, 80% kernels	34	30	7
Hamburger bun	61	30	9
Kaiser roll	73	30	12
Pumpernickel bread	56	30	7
50% cracked wheat kernel bread	58	30	12
White wheat flour bread, average	75	30	11
Wonder® bread, average	73	30	10

Whole wheat bread, average	69	30	9
100% Whole Grain® bread (Natural Ovens)	51	30	7
Pita bread, white	68	30	10

Corn tortilla	52	50	12
Wheat tortilla	30	50	8
BEVERAGES			
Coca Cola® (US formula)	63	250 mL	16
Fanta®, orange soft drink	68	250 mL	23
Lucozade®, original (sparkling glucose drink)	95	250 mL	40
Apple juice, unsweetened,	41	250 mL	12
Cranberry juice cocktail (Ocean Spray®)	68	250 mL	24
Gatorade, orange flavor (US formula)	89	250 mL	13
Orange juice, unsweetened, average	50	250 mL	12
Tomato juice, canned, no sugar added	38	250 mL	4
BREAKFAST CEREALS AND RELATED PRODUCTS			
All-Bran®, average	44	30	9
Coco Pops®, average	77	30	20
Cornflakes®, average	81	30	20
Cream of Wheat®	66	250	17
Cream of Wheat®, Instant	74	250	22

Grape-Nuts®	75	30	16
Muesli, average	56	30	10
Oatmeal, average	55	250	13
Instant oatmeal, average	79	250	21
Puffed wheat cereal	80	30	17
Raisin Bran®	61	30	12
Special K® (US formula)	69	30	14

GRAINS			
Pearled barley, average	25	150	11
Sweet corn on the cob	48	60	14
Couscous	65	150	9
Quinoa	53	150	13
White rice, average	73	150	43
Quick cooking white basmati	63	150	26
Brown rice, average	68	150	16
Parboiled Converted white rice (Uncle Ben's®)	38	150	14
Whole wheat kernels, average	45	50	15
Bulgur, average	47	150	12
COOKIES AND CRACKERS			
Graham crackers	74	25	13
Vanilla wafers	77	25	14

Shortbread	64	25	10
Rice cakes, average	82	25	17
Rye crisps, average	64	25	11
Soda crackers	74	25	12
DAIRY PRODUCTS AND ALTERNATIVES			
Ice cream, regular, average	62	50	8
Ice cream, premium (Sara Lee®)	38	50	3
Milk, full-fat, average	31	250 mL	4
Milk, skim, average	31	250 mL	4
Reduced-fat yogurt with fruit, average	33	200	11

FRUITS			
Apple, average	36	120	5
Banana, raw, average	48	120	11
Dates, dried, average	42	60	18
Grapefruit	25	120	3
Grapes, black	59	120	11
Oranges, raw, average	45	120	45
Peach, average	42	120	5
Peach, canned in light syrup	52	120	9
Pear, raw, average	38	120	4
Pear, canned in pear juice	44	120	5

Prunes, pitted	29	60	10
Raisins	64	60	28
Watermelon	72	120	4
BEANS AND NUTS			
Baked beans	40	150	6
Black-eyed peas	50	150	15
Black beans	30	150	7
Chickpeas	10	150	3
Chickpeas, canned in brine	42	150	9
Navy beans, average	39	150	12
Kidney beans, average	34	150	9
Lentils	28	150	5
Soy beans, average	15	150	1

Cashews, salted	22	50	3
Peanuts	13	50	1
PASTA and NOODLES			
Fettucini	32	180	15
Macaroni, average	50	180	24
Macaroni and Cheese (Kraft®)	64	180	33
Spaghetti, white, boiled, average	46	180	22
Spaghetti, white, boiled 20 min	58	180	26

Spaghetti, whole-grain, boiled	42	180	17
SNACK FOODS			
Corn chips, plain, salted, average	42	50	11
Fruit Roll-Ups®	99	30	24
M & M's®, peanut	33	30	6
Microwave popcorn, plain, average	55	20	7
Potato chips, average	56	50	12
Pretzels, oven-baked	83	30	16
Snickers Bar®	51	60	18
VEGETABLES			
Green peas	54	80	4
Carrots, average	39	80	2
Parsnips	52	80	4
Baked russet potato	111	150	33
Boiled white potato, average	82	150	21
Instant mashed potato, average	87	150	17
Sweet potato, average	70	150	22
Yam, average	54	150	20
MISCELLANEOUS			
Hummus (chickpea salad dip)	6	30	0
Chicken nuggets, frozen, reheated in microwave oven 5 min	46	100	7
Honey, average	61	25	12

NOVICE WORKOUT LOG

Date:

_____

Start Time: _____

Week: _____

Rate of Breath: _____

End Time: _____

Track your fitness progress

Day 1:

After the |, record the number of repetitions completed.

Workout	Warm up	Weight	Set 1	Set 2	Set 3	Set 4
Example			10 | <u>8</u>	10 | <u>10</u>	10 | <u>9</u>	
Hyperextension	None		10 |	10 |	10 |	
Bench Press	Yes		5 |	5 |	5 |	5 |
Deadlifts	Yes		5 |	5 |	5 |	5 |
Barbell Squat	Yes		5 |	5 |	5 |	5 |
Seated Calf Raises	None		6 |	6 |	6 |	
Leg Lifts & Stability Ball Crunches	None		F |	F |	F |	

Day 2:

Workout	Warm up	Weight	Set 1	Set 2	Set 3	Set 4
Hyperextension	None		10 |	10 |	10 |	
Bench Press	Yes		5 |	5 |	5 |	5 |
Deadlifts	Yes		5 |	5 |	5 |	5 |
Barbell Squat	Yes		5 |	5 |	5 |	5 |
Seated Calf Raises	None		15 |	15 |	15 |	
Leg Lifts & Stability Ball Crunches	None		F |	F |	F |	

Day 3:

Workout	Warm up	Weight	Set 1	Set 2	Set 3	Set 4
Hyperextension	None		10 |	10 |	10 |	
Bench Press	Yes		5 |	5 |	5 |	5 |
Deadlifts	Yes		5 |	5 |	5 |	5 |
Barbell Squat	Yes		5 |	5 |	5 |	5 |
Seated Calf Raises	None		6 |	6 |	6 |	
Leg Lifts & Stability Ball Crunches	None		F |	F |	F |	

Date: _____   Start Time: _____

Week: _____

Rate of Breath: _____

End Time: _____

Track your fitness progress

Day 1:

After the |, record the number of repetitions completed.

If you can do more than 5 reps per set, up the weight. If you cannot do more than 3 reps, lower the weight

Workout	Weight	Set 1	Set 2	Set 3	Set 4	Set 5
Example		10 | <u>8</u>	10 | <u>8</u>	10 | <u>10</u>		
Hyperextension		10 |	10 |	10 |		
Barbell Squat		5 |	5 |	5 |	5 |	5 |
Bench press		5 |	5 |	5 |	5 |	5 |
Standing Barbell Press		5 |	5 |	5 |	5 |	5 |
Upright Row		5 |	5 |	5 |	5 |	5 |
Deadlift		5 |	5 |	5 |	5 |	5 |
Standing Calf Raise		25 |	25 |	25 |		
Leg Raises & Reverse Crunches		F |	F |	F |		

Day 2:

Workout	Weight	Set 1	Set 2	Set 3	Set 4	Set 5
Hyperextension		10 |	10 |	10 |		
Barbell Squat		5 |	5 |	5 |	5 |	5 |
Bench press		5 |	5 |	5 |	5 |	5 |
Standing Barbell Press		5 |	5 |	5 |	5 |	5 |
Upright Row		5 |	5 |	5 |	5 |	5 |
Deadlift		5 |	5 |	5 |	5 |	5 |
Standing Calf Raise		25 |	25 |	25 |		
Leg Raises & Reverse Crunches		F |	F |	F |		

Day 3:

Workout	Weight	Set 1	Set 2	Set 3	Set 4	Set 5
Hyperextension		10 |	10 |	10 |		
Workout	**Weight**	**Set 1**	**Set 2**	**Set 3**	**Set 4**	**Set 5**
Barbell Squat		5 |	5 |	5 |	5 |	5 |
Bench press		5 |	5 |	5 |	5 |	5 |

Standing Barbell Press		5		5		5		5		5	
Upright Row		5		5		5		5		5	
Deadlift		5		5		5		5		5	
Standing Calf Raise		25		25		25			
Leg Raises & Reverse Crunches		F		F		F			

HERCULEAN WORKOUT LOG

Date: _____   Start Time: _____

Week: _____

Rate of Breath: _____

End Time : _____

Track your fitness progress

Day 1:

After the |, record the number of repetitions completed.

If you can achieve over 10 reps, up the weight by 5lb's. If you can't do 6, lower the weight.

Workout	Weight	Set 1	Set 2	Set 3
Example		8-12 | <u>8</u>	8-12 | <u>8</u>	8-12 | <u>10</u>
Upright Rows		8-12 |	8-12 |	8-12 |
Bench Press		8-12 |	8-12 |	8-12 |
Bent Over Barbell Row		8-12 |	8-12 |	8-12 |
Dumbbell Laterals		8-12 |	8-12 |	8-12 |
Incline press		8-12 |	8-12 |	8-12 |
Dips		8-12 |	8-12 |	8-12 |
Barbell Curls		8-12 |	8-12 |	8-12 |
Standing Dumbbell Curls		8-12 |	8-12 |	8-12 |
Dumbbell Pullovers		8-12 |	8-12 |	8-12 |
Squats		8-12 |	8-12 |	8-12 |
Deadlifts		8-12 |	8-12 |	8-12 |
Hyperextensions		8-12 |	8-12 |	
Calf Extensions		15 |	15 |	15 |
Leg Lifts & Stability Ball Crunches		F |	F |	F |

Day 2:

Workout	Weight	Set 1	Set 2	Set 3
Upright Rows		8-12 |	8-12 |	8-12 |
Bench Press		8-12 |	8-12 |	8-12 |
Bent Over Barbell Row		8-12 |	8-12 |	8-12 |
Dumbbell Laterals		8-12 |	8-12 |	8-12 |
Incline press		8-12 |	8-12 |	8-12 |
Dips		8-12 |	8-12 |	8-12 |
Barbell Curls		8-12 |	8-12 |	8-12 |
Standing Dumbbell Curls		8-12 |	8-12 |	8-12 |
Dumbbell Pullovers		8-12 |	8-12 |	8-12 |
Squats		8-12 |	8-12 |	8-12 |

Workout	Weight	Set 1	Set 2	Set 3
Deadlifts		8-12 |	8-12 |	8-12 |
Hyperextensions		8-12 |	8-12 |	
Calf Extensions		15 |	15 |	15 |
Leg Lifts & Stability Ball Crunches		F |	F |	F |

Day 3:

Workout	Weight	Set 1	Set 2	Set 3
Upright Rows		8-12 |	8-12 |	8-12 |
Bench Press		8-12 |	8-12 |	8-12 |
Bent Over Barbell Row		8-12 |	8-12 |	8-12 |
Dumbbell Laterals		8-12 |	8-12 |	8-12 |
Incline press		8-12 |	8-12 |	8-12 |
Dips		8-12 |	8-12 |	8-12 |
Barbell Curls		8-12 |	8-12 |	8-12 |
Standing Dumbbell Curls		8-12 |	8-12 |	8-12 |
Dumbbell Pullovers		8-12 |	8-12 |	8-12 |
Squats		8-12 |	8-12 |	8-12 |
Deadlifts		8-12 |	8-12 |	8-12 |
Hyperextensions		8-12 |	8-12 |	
Calf Extensions		15 |	15 |	15 |
Leg Lifts & Stability Ball Crunches		F |	F |	F |

DESERTER WORKOUT LOG

Date: _____   Start Time: _____

Week: _____

Rate of Breath: _____

End Time: _____

Track your fitness progress

Day 1:

After the |, record the number of repetitions completed.

Workout	Weight	Set 1	Set 2	Set 3	Set 4	Set 5
Example		10 | <u>8</u>	10 | <u>8</u>	10 | <u>10</u>		
Hyperextension		10 |	10 |	10 |		
Front squat		8 |	8 |	8 |		
Squat		6 |	6 |	6 |	6 |	
Romanian Deadlift		8 |	8 |	8 |		
Standing Barbell Press		8 |	8 |	8 |	8 |	8 |
Standing Lateral Raises		10 |	10 |	10 |	10 |	
Bench Press		5 |	5 |	5 |	5 |	
Incline Barbell Press		8 |	8 |	8 |	8 |	
Pull-up		8 |	8 |	8 |	8 |	8 |
Barbell Row		8 |	8 |	8 |		
Barbell Curl		8 |	8 |	8 |	8 |	
Dips		8 |	8 |	8 |	8 |	
Standing Barbell Calf Raise		25 |	25 |	25 |		
Standing Calf Raise		25 |	25 |	25 |		
Leg Raises & Reverse Crunches		F |	F |	F |		

Day 2:

Workout	Weight	Set 1	Set 2	Set 3	Set 4	Set 5
Hyperextension		10 |	10 |	10 |		
Front squat		8 |	8 |	8 |		
Squat		6 |	6 |	6 |	6 |	
Romanian Deadlift		8 |	8 |	8 |		
Standing Barbell Press		8 |	8 |	8 |	8 |	8 |

Standing Lateral Raises		10		10		10		10		
Bench Press		5		5		5		5		
Incline Barbell Press		8		8		8		8		
Pull-up		8		8		8		8		8	
Barbell Row		8		8		8			
Barbell Curl		8		8		8		8		
Dips		8		8		8		8		
Standing Barbell Calf Raise		25		25		25			
Standing Calf Raises		25		25		25			
Leg Raises & Reverse Crunches		F		F		F			

Day 3:

Workout	Weight	Set 1	Set 2	Set 3	Set 4	Set 5
Hyperextension		10		10		10			
Front squat		8		8		8			
Squat		6		6		6		6		
Romanian Deadlift		8		8		8			
Standing Barbell Press		8		8		8		8		8	
Standing Lateral Raises		10		10		10		10		
Bench Press		5		5		5		5		
Incline Barbell Press		8		8		8		8		

Pull-up		8 |	8 |	8 |	8 |	8 |
Barbell Row		8 |	8 |	8 |		
Barbell Curl		8 |	8 |	8 |	8 |	
Dips		8 |	8 |	8 |	8 |	
Standing Barbell Calf Raise		25 |	25 |	25 |		
Standing Calf Raise		25 |	25 |	25 |		

Leg Raises & Reverse Crunches		F |	F |	F |		

For More Information or Tailored Training Email

shane@bodyengineering.com